A Summary of the October 2009
Forum on the Future of Nursing

ACUTE CARE

Committee on the Robert Wood Johnson
Foundation Initiative on the Future of Nursing,
at the Institute of Medicine

INSTITUTE OF MEDICINE
OF THE NATIONAL ACADEMIES

THE NATIONAL ACADEMIES PRESS
Washington, D.C.
www.nap.edu

THE NATIONAL ACADEMIES PRESS • 500 Fifth Street, N.W. • Washington, DC 20001

NOTICE: The project that is the subject of this report was approved by the Governing Board of the National Research Council, whose members are drawn from the councils of the National Academy of Sciences, the National Academy of Engineering, and the Institute of Medicine. The members of the committee responsible for the report were chosen for their special competences and with regard for appropriate balance.

Support for this project was provided by the Robert Wood Johnson Foundation (Contract No. 65815). Any opinions, findings, conclusions, or recommendations expressed in this publication are those of the author(s) and do not necessarily reflect the views of the organizations or agencies that provided support for the project.

International Standard Book Number-13: 978-0-309-15021-7
International Standard Book Number-10: 0-309-15021-3

Additional copies of this report are available from the National Academies Press, 500 Fifth Street, N.W., Lockbox 285, Washington, DC 20055; (800) 624-6242 or (202) 334-3313 (in the Washington metropolitan area); Internet, http://www.nap.edu.

For more information about the Institute of Medicine, visit the IOM home page at: **www.iom.edu.**

Printed in the United States of America

Cover credit: Select photos reprinted with permission from Lisa Hollis of Cedars-Sinai Medical Center.

Suggested citation: IOM (Institute of Medicine). 2010. *A summary of the October 2009 forum on the future of nursing: Acute care.* Washington, DC: The National Academies Press.

*"Knowing is not enough; we must apply.
Willing is not enough; we must do."*
—Goethe

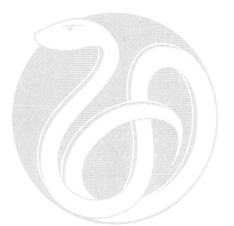

INSTITUTE OF MEDICINE
OF THE NATIONAL ACADEMIES

Advising the Nation. Improving Health.

THE NATIONAL ACADEMIES
Advisers to the Nation on Science, Engineering, and Medicine

The **National Academy of Sciences** is a private, nonprofit, self-perpetuating society of distinguished scholars engaged in scientific and engineering research, dedicated to the furtherance of science and technology and to their use for the general welfare. Upon the authority of the charter granted to it by the Congress in 1863, the Academy has a mandate that requires it to advise the federal government on scientific and technical matters. Dr. Ralph J. Cicerone is president of the National Academy of Sciences.

The **National Academy of Engineering** was established in 1964, under the charter of the National Academy of Sciences, as a parallel organization of outstanding engineers. It is autonomous in its administration and in the selection of its members, sharing with the National Academy of Sciences the responsibility for advising the federal government. The National Academy of Engineering also sponsors engineering programs aimed at meeting national needs, encourages education and research, and recognizes the superior achievements of engineers. Dr. Charles M. Vest is president of the National Academy of Engineering.

The **Institute of Medicine** was established in 1970 by the National Academy of Sciences to secure the services of eminent members of appropriate professions in the examination of policy matters pertaining to the health of the public. The Institute acts under the responsibility given to the National Academy of Sciences by its congressional charter to be an adviser to the federal government and, upon its own initiative, to identify issues of medical care, research, and education. Dr. Harvey V. Fineberg is president of the Institute of Medicine.

The **National Research Council** was organized by the National Academy of Sciences in 1916 to associate the broad community of science and technology with the Academy's purposes of furthering knowledge and advising the federal government. Functioning in accordance with general policies determined by the Academy, the Council has become the principal operating agency of both the National Academy of Sciences and the National Academy of Engineering in providing services to the government, the public, and the scientific and engineering communities. The Council is administered jointly by both Academies and the Institute of Medicine. Dr. Ralph J. Cicerone and Dr. Charles M. Vest are chair and vice chair, respectively, of the National Research Council.

www.national-academies.org

COMMITTEE ON THE ROBERT WOOD JOHNSON FOUNDATION INITIATIVE ON THE FUTURE OF NURSING, AT THE INSTITUTE OF MEDICINE

DONNA E. SHALALA (*Chair*), University of Miami, Coral Gables, FL
LINDA BURNES BOLTON (*Vice Chair*), Cedars-Sinai Health System and Research Institute, Los Angeles, CA
MICHAEL BLEICH, Oregon Health & Science University School of Nursing, Portland
TROYEN A. BRENNAN, CVS Caremark, Woonsocket, RI
ROBERT E. CAMPBELL, Johnson & Johnson (*retired*), New Brunswick, NJ
LEAH DEVLIN, University of North Carolina at Chapel Hill, School of Public Health
CATHERINE DOWER, University of California–San Francisco
ROSA GONZALEZ-GUARDA, University of Miami, Coral Gables, FL
DAVID C. GOODMAN, Dartmouth Medical School, Hanover, NH
JENNIE CHIN HANSEN, AARP, Washington, DC
C. MARTIN HARRIS, Cleveland Clinic, Cleveland, OH
ANJLI AURORA HINMAN, Intown Midwifery, Atlanta, GA
WILLIAM D. NOVELLI, Georgetown University, Washington, DC
LIANA ORSOLINI-HAIN, City College of San Francisco, CA
YOLANDA PARTIDA, University of California–San Francisco, Fresno
ROBERT D. REISCHAUER, Urban Institute, Washington, DC
JOHN W. ROWE, Columbia University, New York
BRUCE C. VLADECK, Nexera Consulting, New York

Study Staff
JUDITH A. SALERNO, Executive Officer
SUSAN HASSMILLER, Director, Robert Wood Johnson Foundation Initiative on the Future of Nursing, at the Institute of Medicine
ADRIENNE STITH BUTLER, Senior Program Officer
ANDREA M. SCHULTZ, Associate Program Officer
KATHARINE BOTHNER, Research Associate
THELMA L. COX, Administrative Assistant
TONIA E. DICKERSON, Senior Program Assistant
GINA IVEY, Communications Director, Robert Wood Johnson Foundation Initiative on the Future of Nursing, at the Institute of Medicine

LORI MELICHAR, Research Director, Robert Wood Johnson Foundation Initiative on the Future of Nursing, at the Institute of Medicine
JULIE FAIRMAN, Nurse Scholar-in-Residence

Consultants
PAUL LIGHT, New York University
STEVE OLSON, Technical Writer
JOSEF REUM, The George Washington University, Washington, DC

Reviewers

This report has been reviewed in draft form by individuals chosen for their diverse perspectives and technical expertise, in accordance with procedures approved by the National Research Council's Report Review Committee. The purpose of this independent review is to provide candid and critical comments that will assist the institution in making its published report as sound as possible and to ensure that the report meets institutional standards for objectivity, evidence, and responsiveness to the study charge. The review comments and draft manuscript remain confidential to protect the integrity of the process. We wish to thank the following individuals for their review of this report:

Suzanne M. Boyle, New York Presbyterian Weill Cornell Hospital
Larry A. Green, University of Colorado at Denver
Angela Barron McBride, Indiana University School of Nursing
Alan H. Rosenstein, Physician Wellness Services

Although the reviewers listed above have provided many constructive comments and suggestions, they were not asked to endorse the final draft of the report before its release. The review of this report was overseen by **Ada Sue Hinshaw,** Graduate School of Nursing, Uniformed Services University of the Health Sciences. Appointed by the National Research Council and the Institute of Medicine, she was responsible for making certain that an independent examination of this report was carried out in accordance with institutional procedures and that all review comments were carefully considered. Responsibility for the final content of this report rests entirely with the authors and the institution.

Preface

On October 19, 2009, the Cedars-Sinai Medical Center hosted the first of three public forums of the Initiative on the Future of Nursing, a collaborative effort between the Robert Wood Johnson Foundation (RWJF) and the Institute of Medicine (IOM). In the morning, several members of the IOM committee toured a number of the Center's acute care units to experience firsthand the innovations in nursing pioneered at Cedars-Sinai. In the afternoon, more than 300 people attended the forum—and hundreds more from across the United States watched on a live webcast—to hear approximately 30 speakers explore new approaches that involve nurses providing safe, efficient, and effective care in acute care settings and across the health continuum. In the evening, about 30 RWJF scholars and fellows, who also attended the forum and the morning's site visits, dug more deeply into the issues to develop their recommendations for the future of nursing in acute care settings. The day was intense, exhilarating, and extremely productive.

Many unknowns about health care remain as the country pushes ahead with health care reform. But one thing is certain: The United States cannot adequately address the challenges facing its health care system without also addressing the challenges facing the nursing profession. Nurses are the largest segment of the health care workforce and are essential to providing quality care. Yet projected shortages of nurses, a lack of opportunities for educational advancement, limited resources, and the fragmented environment in which nurses provide care pose formidable barriers to fulfilling the promise of health care reform. The goal of the Initiative is to help transform nursing as part of far-reaching reforms in the health care system.

The forum was an information-gathering session that the committee used to hear perspectives and ideas, which it will examine in depth and discuss as it shapes its findings, conclusions, and recommendations. This summary of the forum presents the main points made by invited speakers, panelists, and forum participants who offered testimony at its conclusion. The summary should not be seen as representing the positions of committee members in attendance, the IOM, RWJF, or the Cedars-Sinai Medical Center. Committee members typically ask probing questions in information-gathering sessions such as forums, and these questions may not be indicative of their personal views. In addition, under the skilled direction of the forum's moderator, Dr. Josef Reum, interim dean of the School of Public Health and Health Services at the George Washington University, committee members, speakers, and participants at the forum explored a broad array of issues and perspectives on the many challenges that face nursing.

The forum focused on three topics within the context of acute care: safety, technology, and interdisciplinary collaboration. A number of important points emerged at the forum, but the ones that resonated with our experiences include the following:

- The knowledge of frontline nurses that they gather from their interactions with patients is critical to reducing medical errors and improving patient outcomes.
- Involving nurses at a variety of levels across the acute care setting in decision making and leadership benefits the patient, improves the organizations in which nurses practice, and strengthens the health care system in general.
- Increasing the time that nurses can spend at the bedside is an essential component of achieving the goal of patient-centered care.
- High-quality acute care settings require integrated systems that use technology effectively while increasing the efficiency of nurses and affording them increased time to spend with patients.
- Multidisciplinary care teams characterized by extensive and respectful collaboration among team members improve the quality, safety, and effectiveness of care.
- Many of the innovations that need to be implemented in the health care system already exist somewhere in the United States, but barriers to their dissemination keep them from being adopted more widely. As Dr. Marilyn Chow observed, "the future is here, it just isn't everywhere."

The current system of health care in the United States is unsustainable. Now is our chance to get the system on a sustainable and productive path by looking to the mistakes of the past and alternative remedies for the future. The IOM committee, which is chaired by University of Miami President Dr. Donna Shalala, is developing a set of bold recommendations and a clear agenda for action. It is considering changes in public and institutional policies at the federal, state, and local levels as it seeks to provide guidance on the future of nursing.

Nurses have the benefit of experience in identifying problems and the capability to implement solutions that work for patients. To achieve the promise of health care reform, we need to keep the better parts of our current health care system and eliminate the less effective parts that are not adding value. The Initiative on the Future of Nursing is an important step toward making that goal a reality.

Linda Burnes Bolton
Committee Vice Chair and Forum Host

Robert D. Reischauer
Committee Member and Forum Planning Group Chair

Acknowledgments

The Robert Wood Johnson Foundation (RWJF) Initiative on the Future of Nursing, at the Institute of Medicine (IOM), wishes to thank the many individuals and organizations that contributed to the *Forum on the Future of Nursing: Acute Care*. The forum was graciously hosted by Linda Burnes Bolton and Tom Priselac at Cedars-Sinai Medical Center. Their staff, particularly Barbara Fields, Lynette Huff, and Jane Swanson, ensured seamless arrangements for the day, including several site visits to various units of the Medical Center. The Initiative would also like to thank the speakers, panelists, and all who provided testimony throughout the plenary sessions; the insight and experience that was shared with the committee contributed greatly to its deliberations.

The sessions were facilitated by Josef Reum, broadcast online by ON24, and transcribed by Joy Biletz. The Initiative is grateful to Steve Olson for his editorial and writing assistance, to Laura Penny for copyediting the summary, and to Dan Banks for designing the cover.

The forum would not have been a success without the willingness of the committee planning group to lend their time and expertise. The planning group was chaired by Robert Reischauer, and included Linda Burnes Bolton, Catherine Dower, Rosa Gonzalez-Guarda, David Goodman, Martin Harris, Anjli Aurora Hinman, Liana Orsolini-Hain, and Yolanda Partida.

Following the forum, a group of alumni from various RWJF fellow and scholar programs gathered to reflect on the day's discussions. They proposed several thoughtful and innovative ideas for the future of nursing in the acute care setting to the committee.

For their diligent and creative work throughout the course of the forum, we would like to recognize the Initiative staff members, led by

Susan Hassmiller and Adrienne Stith Butler, with guidance and oversight from Judith Salerno. The following individuals were involved in planning the forum, day-of support, and the production of this summary: Katharine Bothner, Thelma Cox, Julie Dashiell, Tonia Dickerson, Gina Ivey, Lori Melichar, Abbey Meltzer, and Andrea Schultz. We would also like to recognize the contributions of the following staff and consultants to this activity: Clyde Behney, Julie Fairman, Christine Gorman, Jillian Grady, Amy Levey, Paul Light, Sharon Reis, Autumn Rose, Christine Stencel, Vilija Teel, Lauren Tobias, Jackie Turner, Gary Walker, and Jordan Wyndelts.

Finally, the Initiative would like to express its appreciation to RWJF, whose generous financial support, and mission to improve the health and health care of all Americans, made the forum possible.

Contents

APPENDIXES

1

Introduction

On October 19, 2009, the Initiative on the Future of Nursing, a collaborative effort between the Robert Wood Johnson Foundation (RWJF) and the Institute of Medicine (IOM), held a forum at Cedars-Sinai Medical Center in Los Angeles to examine the challenges facing the nursing profession and the changes needed in nursing to improve the quality, efficiency, and effectiveness of patient care. The forum was the first of three and focused on the future of nursing in acute care settings. The second forum, on December 3, 2009, in Philadelphia, looked at nursing care in the community, with emphasis on community health, public health, primary care, and long-term care. The third forum, on February 22, 2010, in Houston, examined the future of nursing education.

The three half-day forums were not meant to be an exhaustive examination of all settings where nurses practice nor an exhaustive examination of the complexity of the nursing profession as a whole. Given the limited amount of time for each of the three forums, a comprehensive review of all facets and all players of each of the main forum themes was not possible. Rather, the forums were meant to inform the committee on important topics within the nursing profession and highlight some of the key challenges, barriers, opportunities, and innovations that nurses face while working in an evolving health care system. Many key challenges, barriers, opportunities, and innovations discussed at the forums overlap across settings and throughout the nursing profession. They are also applicable to other providers and individuals who work with nurses.

The forums have been part of an intensive information-gathering effort by an IOM committee that is the cornerstone of the Initiative on the Future of Nursing. The committee will use the information collected at these forums, at its two technical workshops, from data provided by the

RWJF Nursing Research Network, and from a number of commissioned papers to inform the development of findings, conclusions, and recommendations. The committee's final recommendations will be presented in a report on the capacity of the nursing workforce to meet the demands of a reformed health care system.

This summary of the forum describes the main points made by speakers and participants throughout the afternoon session in Los Angeles. A complete agenda of the forum can be found in Appendix B and biosketches for the speakers can be found in Appendix C. The remaining sections of this chapter describe two activities that occurred in conjunction with the forum and present the introduction to the forum by Thomas Priselac, president and chief executive officer of the Cedars-Sinai Health System and chair of the Board of Directors for the American Hospital Association. Chapter 2 provides an overview of the issues facing acute care nurses, as presented by Dr. Marilyn Chow, vice president of National Patient Care Services at Kaiser Permanente in Oakland, CA. Chapters 3 through 5 are organized by the three main topics discussed at the forum: the quality and safety of care, technology, and interdisciplinary collaboration. These chapters include the summaries of the presentations, reactions from the panelists, and the discussion that resulted from the committee's questions and the answers provided by the speakers. Patient care in acute care settings involves a team that includes a spectrum of individuals from nurses to physicians to pharmacists to patients and their families. To hear the diverse, on-the-ground perspectives of some experienced members of the care team, a panel was assembled that consisted of five individuals: an advanced practice nurse, a hospitalist, a pharmacist, a recent nursing student, and a patient. Chapter 6 summarizes the oral testimony presented by 19 forum attendees.

Comments made at the forum should not be interpreted as positions of the committee, RWJF, or IOM. Committee members' questions and comments do not necessarily reflect the conclusions that will be in the committee's report. They were designed to elicit useful and relevant information and perspectives.

SITE VISITS

In the morning before the forum began, individual committee members participated in a series of site visits to a variety of acute care units within Cedars-Sinai Medical Center. They spoke with nurses, other care providers, and administrators about the challenges nurses encounter in their work in acute care settings. Observations made during these site visits are not part of this summary of the forum, but the site visits informed at least some of the questions directed to speakers by committee members at the event. The units that were visited at the hospital ranged from critical care, emergency department, and surgical units to child and maternal health and obstetrics units.

Robert Wood Johnson Foundation Solutions Session

Following the forum, a select group of RWJF scholars and fellows[1] was hosted by RWJF to discuss what they saw on the site visits and heard at the forum in the context of their own expertise, knowledge, and judgment. This session was independent of the IOM committee and the Forum on the Future of Nursing. The goal of this session was to provide an opportunity for the fellows and scholars to consider solutions and the most promising future roles for nurses in the acute care setting with respect to the subthemes of quality and safety, technology, and interdisciplinary collaboration.

The solutions offered by the panels of fellows and scholars are not described in this summary of the forum. But summaries of their solutions were provided to the committee for its review and consideration at the committee's subsequent meeting in November 2009.

FORUM WELCOME

Americans are asking fundamental questions about the future of their health care system, said Thomas Priselac, president and chief executive officer of the Cedars-Sinai Health System, in his opening remarks at the forum. These questions are complex because modern medicine and

---

[1]RWJF works to build human capital by supporting individuals who seek to advance health and health care in America. RWJF invited alumni of seventeen of its scholar, fellow, and leader programs to participate in the Forum on the Future of Nursing. The alumni come from a variety of backgrounds and disciplines, including academia, service delivery, research, policy, and health plan administration. Many of the participants were alumni of the RWJF Executive Nurse Fellows Program and the RWJF Nurse Faculty Scholars Program. Non-nurse participants included alumni of the Investigator Award Program, the RWJF Health Policy Fellows Program, and the RWJF Clinical Scholar Program.

health care are complex. Yet at the core of the health care system is the professional who translates the complexity of modern health care into the unique forms of care focused on and provided to each health care recipient. That person is usually a nurse. "They are, quite simply, the face of health care today," Priselac said.

The American Hospital Association (AHA), which Priselac currently chairs, is committed to improving health care by drawing on the expertise and experiences of nurses and others who provide care in hospitals. About a decade ago, the AHA released a collection of best practices based on programs that enrich and support America's nurses (AHA, 2002). Today many of those practices are standard in hospitals nationwide, he said. "Without effective, trained, satisfied, and engaged nursing, a high-quality care environment is impossible."

What nurses do in today's health care environment must be evaluated regularly to better understand how to support the nurses of tomorrow. The nursing-sensitive performance indicators recently adopted by the Centers for Medicare & Medicaid Services provide an excellent example. These indicators delineate the connections between effective nursing practices and the prevention of avoidable harm, such as injuries from falls, central-line infections, pressure ulcers, and mortality after surgical procedures. Another example of a program that has contributed to understanding the importance of nurses' roles is the Transforming Care at the Bedside (TCAB) initiative, which was supported by RWJF and began in 2003. This nurse-led initiative has demonstrated the many benefits of a strong partnership between nurses and health care executives to improve patient safety and meet quality improvement goals at institutions. Cedars-Sinai Medical Center has been one of 10 innovative hospitals working to make TCAB a national standard, Priselac noted.

Under the leadership of the American Organization of Nurse Executives (AONE), and in collaboration with AHA, TCAB is rapidly becoming an essential part of more and more hospitals' efforts to provide sustainable, reliable, high-quality care every day to everyone, everywhere. In May 2009, AONE announced that TCAB would be at the heart of a new program designed to create the patient care delivery models of the future. Building on a $1.5 million dissemination project funded by RWJF, AONE is expanding the number of participating hospitals. By adding their own experiences to the TCAB initiative, these institutions will contribute to improving the care environment for patients and strengthening the connection between hospital leaders and nurses. The

Institute for Healthcare Improvement, an original TCAB partner, is also disseminating the program.

Nurses represent the largest group of health professionals in the country, Priselac said, and their expertise has a direct effect on the quality, safety, and cost-effectiveness of health care. For example, according to research from the National Quality Forum, the deployment of advanced practice nurses decreases hospital readmissions and improves transitions to nursing homes and community settings. Providing nurses with the knowledge and skills to deliver evidence-based care practices and empowering them to lead in the long-term improvement of health care delivery will be essential in creating a better health care system in the United States.

2

The Current and Future State
of Acute Care

Hospitals are complex and often chaotic places, said Dr. Marilyn Chow, vice president of National Patient Care Services at Kaiser Permanente in Oakland, CA. This complexity is due in part to the nature of patients' conditions. But it also arises from technologies that are not seamlessly connected to each other, including electronic health records (EHRs), biomedical devices, and robotic devices.

Nurses are the primary professional caregivers in hospitals. The efficient use of their time and energy is critical to the functioning of hospitals and acute care. Yet nurses' time is not used efficiently today. According to a study led by Chow and Ann Hendrich, vice president of Clinical Excellence Operations for Ascension Health in St. Louis, of 767 nurses at 36 medical surgery units, the tasks of medication administration, care coordination, and documentation consumed the majority of all nursing practice time—part of an estimated $50 billion spent on documentation in health care annually. As shown in Figure 2-1, less than one fifth of nursing practice time went to direct patient care activities, such as providing procedures and treatments at the bedside. Just 7.2 percent of nursing time was spent on patient assessment and vital signs. "That equates to about 31 minutes out of each 10-hour shift," Chow observed (Hendrich et al., 2008).

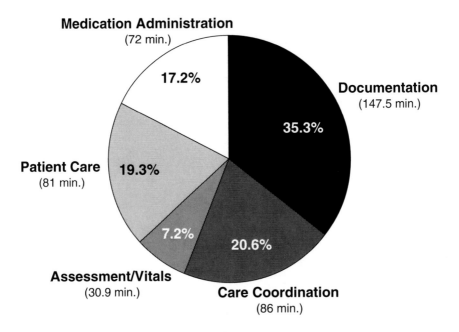

FIGURE 2-1 How do nurses spend their time?
SOURCE: Hendrich et al. (2008). Reprinted from *The Permanente Journal*, (www.kp.org/permanentejournal) 12(3), Hendrich, A., M. Chow, B. A. Skierczynski, and Z. Lu, A time and motion study: How do medical-surgical nurses spend their time?, 37-46, copyright 2008, reprinted with permission from The Permanente Press.

The working conditions of nurses are extremely stressful. They often deliver care within inefficient and disconnected systems; they manage a complex list of physician orders that require continuous reprioritizing; they perform the critical functions of surveillance and continuous monitoring of patients; and they do this work while "hunting and gathering" for equipment, supplies, and personnel, and experiencing frequent interruptions and distractions. They become what Chow called "masters of work-arounds" for systems that do not function well.

Over the next decade, Chow asserted, new practice models are needed "that focus on the real contributions of nurses, and we need to change the way we organize and deliver that care." For example, the Gordon and Betty Moore Foundation has funded a project called Destination Bedside in two Kaiser facilities in Northern California. It is seeking to create more effective work environments that seamlessly support nurses and other clinicians in the delivery of patient care. In addition, a variety of recent articles, reports, and books have brought new thinking and new ideas to the practice of nursing from both within and outside of health care.

Chow said she has spent a lot of time listening to people about their hospital experiences and asking them what was missing, what could be done differently, and what made a difference in their experiences. She has found that information and knowledge are growing "at warp speed." The acute care environment is being reshaped by technologies, new business models, and human needs. New acute care models will either emerge haphazardly by default or coherently by design. Furthermore, aspects of some coherent new models are already evident in the health care system. "The future is already here. It's just not everywhere."

CORE CONCEPTS FOR IMAGINING THE FUTURE OF NURSING

Chow focused on five core concepts, described below, for imagining the future of nursing in acute care.

Core Concept 1: Leverage the Power of the Electronic Health Record

The EHR could be the connective tissue of the health care system. An EHR not bound to one site or caregiver could enable improved care coordination and transitions, provide complete information connectivity, and transform the manner in which care is delivered and received, Chow said.

Kaiser Permanente has learned many lessons from the electronic system it has developed and implemented. Last year the system had 6 million electronic visits—"imagine the personal time savings for the patient, having an e-visit, versus coming into a clinic or an emergency department," Chow said. The EHR has enabled the invention of new patient-centered roles for nurses. For example, a pilot program in a Southern California Kaiser Permanente emergency department called the "Virtual Charge Nurse" tracks patients from the time they arrive at a hospital until a decision is made to discharge or admit them. The EHR shows what has or has not happened to a patient, allowing tests and procedures to be moved online and providing patients with a "virtual advocate." In another program, EHRs have been used to standardize the documentation and management of pressure ulcers. In Kaiser's experience, the implementation of EHRs has reduced documentation loads and increased nurses' time in patient rooms. "The EHR is a tool that will raise the bar for care delivery across all settings, including acute care," said Chow. "It must be seamlessly integrated with other technologies and devices so that nurses are not the human interface for technology that does not work together."

Core Concept 2: Achieve a Balance Among Technologies, Disruptive Business Models, and Human Needs

Incredible technological developments are on the horizon. For example, Chow highlighted miniaturization and wireless technologies that are being used to create body sensor networks that will monitor everything from heartbeats to brainwaves to temperature to blood glucose levels from anywhere in the hospital or even remotely from home.

The convergence of molecular biology, computer, and medical science with electrical, mechanical, genetic, and biomedical engineering could have profound effects on practice models. In a revolutionized future, technologies could assist nurses with much of their work and help consumers in diagnosing and treating themselves with self-help tools and personalized designer drugs. An example is the website developed by Microsoft and Emory University (www.h1n1responsecenter.com) that allows users to determine if they likely have the flu, whether or not to be seen by a health care provider, and what their overall risk is as a flu patient. "Imagine smart systems to guide patients and clinicians through available health information," Chow said. Such technologies produce what she called a "wow factor."

So-called disruptive innovations and business models,[1] such as retail health care clinics, nurse navigators, health coaches, and patient advocates, could be another prominent feature of a future health care system. These disruptive business models could have a major impact on nursing practice. Furthermore, these innovations can be combined with or en-

---

[1]A "disruptive innovation" has been defined by Clayton Christensen as "a process by which a product or service takes root initially in simple applications at the bottom of a market and then relentlessly moves 'up market,' eventually displacing established competitors. An innovation that is disruptive allows a whole new population of consumers access to a product or service that was historically only accessible to consumers with a lot of money or a lot of skill" (Christensen, 1997, 2009).

abled by technology. In the future, technology will come to people rather than people going to the technology. "Remember when you had to send your printing requests to a central duplication center?" Chow asked. "Now you can print at your own desk." In 2002, for example, General Electric sold a conventional ultrasound machine for $100,000 and up to sophisticated hospital imaging centers. In 2007, GE sold a portable ultrasound machine for emerging markets in developing countries at a price of $15,000, giving remote areas access to high technology.

Disruptive innovations aimed directly at human needs have been far less plentiful. "What would we [need to] do to actually be human centered? What are the core human needs? Is it that I hate to travel to the doctor's office or the emergency department, but that I still want someone to look me in the eye, to listen to me, to touch my hand, and to advocate for me? How might we design for human needs and more efficiency, while using innovative business-to-business and technology tools?" The goal is to find a balance among technology, disruptive innovations, and human needs.

Core Concepts 3 and 4: Implement Rapid Translation Teams and Interdisciplinary Teams of Designers

Nurses cannot design a patient-centered system by themselves. Technologies are arriving faster than they can be integrated into the health care system, and people are not able to make sense of much of the information already available. Chow suggested that one possible solution to this deluge of new technology and information is the creation of rapid translation teams. They would assist in the implementation of patient-centered systems that were developed by interdisciplinary teams of designers.

These rapid translation teams could scan, understand, and integrate the technological environment and make connections among technology, research, science, and acute care. Teams could include nurses and other experts such as engineers, geneticists, academic researchers, architects, ethnographers, designers, technologists, change specialists, and frontline clinicians. Rapid translation teams could in turn interact with interdisciplinary teams of designers, including behavioral scientists, marketers, engineers, clinicians, and patients. The result would be a system for designing the future of acute care, with human needs consciously incorporated into the design process. "Change in acute care will happen," Chow said. "It is a question of how we design it."

Core Concept 5: Create an Infrastructure for Rapid Network Exchange of Successful System Design Innovations

A system to design successful innovations will need to be agile. Technological changes occur too quickly to plan, prototype, and test innovations over the course of several years. "We need to create a simple, easy venue for the quick exchange of what's working and not working," Chow explained.

Successful system design innovations also demand leadership and coordination. For example, a national institute for human-centered, empathy-based care with regional nodes could help spread the work of the rapid translation teams and interdisciplinary design teams. Such an institute might focus on economic measures of the value of nursing. It could emphasize an approach to nursing comparable to how one would care for a parent or sibling. "We nurses want to help patients and family members the way we do as the nurses for our families," said Chow. Health innovation design forums could also help disseminate the work of rapid translation and interdisciplinary teams. Nurses could help prototype and pilot new processes, systems, and multidisciplinary practice models.

Several institutions have demonstrated the value of these approaches. For example, the University of Pittsburgh Medical Center has piloted equipment in 22 rooms designed to improve patient safety, increase customer satisfaction, and help nurses and other health care professionals to deliver the right care at the right time, every time. Ascension Health is planning to have three innovation units, and Kaiser Permanente has established a 37,000-square-foot facility to explore the intersection of technology, space, and workflow.

INSTITUTIONAL AND POLICY CHANGES

Nurses have much to learn from other specialties. An example is the role of the nurse navigator in oncology care that could be adapted for use in elder care. Nurses could work to re-purpose solutions found elsewhere. Nurses could also work to generate metrics for face-to-face interactions or system-level measures.

Payment systems need to be changed to recognize the time nurses spend with patients and their families, instead of forcing nurses to squeeze such interactions into their spare time. Chow asked what would need to change from a technology and a systems perspective to make this happen. For example, what if nurses partnered with hospitalists to admit patients? The physician could handle the medical diagnosis and orders while the nurse handles everything else. The nurse could be a single point of contact for the patient and family during a hospital stay as well as during discharge and transition to the home. The nurse could even visit the patient at home, potentially for several months, as happens with Mary Naylor's Transitional Care Model.[2] "We need nurses to think like entrepreneurs and be willing to be designers and experimenters."

Chow also suggested that consideration be given to assigning patients a primary nurse. Patients may have a primary physician and a primary medical assistant. But they do not have a primary nurse.

Federal waivers for state experiments with new practice models could enable expansion of the scope of practice for nurses. In California, for example, a statute enabling health workforce pilot projects has expanded the scope of practice of clinicians beyond current law to test the safety and quality of new, innovative practices. Bringing such waivers to the federal level would allow experimentation that challenges state scope-of-practice laws.

CONCLUSIONS

In Great Britain, Prime Minister Gordon Brown issued the following mandate to the Commission on the Future of Nursing and Midwifery: Reposition nurses and nursing in the eyes of the consumer. That mandate fits with the mission of the Robert Wood Johnson Foundation Initiative on the Future of Nursing, at the Institute of Medicine, Chow said. The chair of the commission, Ann Keen, advised Donna Shalala, the leader of the Initiative on the Future of Nursing, to "have courage, come to the forefront, and stand up for the care you know nurses can do." Chow issued similar advice to the committee: "Timing is everything. Be bold and seize the day."

---

[2]See http://www.transitionalcare.info.

3

Quality and Safety

IMPROVING CARE
THROUGH NURSE EMPOWERMENT

Hospitals strive to provide care that is safe, efficient, effective, patient centered, timely, and equitable, said Maureen Bisognano, executive vice president and chief operating officer at the Institute for Healthcare Improvement (IHI). But variations in safety and quality in hospitals across the United States and worldwide are disquieting, as discussed below:

- *Safety:* Patients in U.S. hospitals experience many preventable adverse drug events. Approximately 90,000 patients die from infections acquired at U.S. hospitals each year, according to the Centers for Disease Control and Prevention (Wenzel and Edmond, 2001). A patient entering a U.S. hospital is about to experience the eighth greatest health hazard in the country, Bisognano said.
- *Effectiveness:* Variations in outcomes from one hospital to the next or even from one unit to another are "too wide for us to accept." There is a failure to identify best practices within a single hospital and share those practices across the units and with multiple hospitals.
- *Efficiency:* Even as hospital costs continue to rise at rates higher than inflation, evidence shows that hospitals with particularly high costs do not necessarily provide higher quality care. Waste is present in most hospitals. It causes delays in care and has both human and financial costs.

- *Patient centeredness:* Many systems and processes are still designed to meet the needs of providers rather than patients. True patient- and family-centered care will focus on the whole patient, putting the patient, family, and care team together as a system.
- *Timeliness:* Delays impose costs not only on hospitals, but on patients in terms of questions unanswered, delayed diagnoses, suffering incurred while waiting for treatments, and lack of coordination. Yet some hospitals have demonstrated that delays in surgeries, for example, can be virtually eliminated. "Our mantra should be: the right care, in the right place, at the right time, in every place in the country," Bisognano said.
- *Inequity:* Continued variations in care delivered and outcomes among socioeconomic and ethnic groups remain unacceptable.

Improvements in the quality of hospital care often occur as a result of national campaigns or programs. By identifying a small number of goals, Bisognano said, such initiatives can work to close gaps among settings. For example, the Commonwealth Fund Commission on a High-Performance Health System has supported the development of a state scorecard on health system performance that has made it possible to translate best practices and knowledge across the system. On a set of hospital clinical quality indicators, the rates in the five lowest performing states approached the previous levels of the highest performing states (McCarthy et al., 2009). "We are starting to see a national awareness of quality and safety and the beginnings of a system to share" best practices and knowledge.

Nurses play a unique role in ensuring quality and safety in hospitals, Bisognano said. "We are the pivot point, we are the people who spend the time, we are the people who see patients across transitions in care." Yet nursing faces many challenges. Care is becoming more complex even as hospital stays become shorter. The nursing population is growing older. The average age of nurses is 44, with many older nurses returning to the workforce in the current economy. Despite the increasing average age of nurses, hospitals are imposing uniform standards and workloads on all nurses. Turnover of nurses is high, shortages of nurses are looming, and nursing staff levels are inadequate in many locations. Finally, nurses still experience an unacceptably high number of work-system failures (an average of 8.4 times per 8-hour shift) and interruptions (an average of 8.1 times per 8-hour shift) (Tucker and Spear, 2006). "Poor system design and the failure to coordinate are going to produce bad results even in the most experienced and savvy nursing staff."

As part of her work at the IHI, Bisognano observes nursing units in hospitals around the world. She described a particular set of innovations at a small community hospital in Cedar Rapids, Iowa, as an example of what can be achieved. When she walked into the hospital, she found a design totally focused on nurses and patients. Everything they need is built into the unit. For example, the dieticians in the hospital are directly linked to the units so they can bring a mobile cart to sit down and counsel patients on their dietary choices. Doctors and nurses make rounds that include not only the patients, but also their families. All family members are welcome to visit patients at any time, and when they walk into a patient's room, the atmosphere is calm and welcoming.

Bisognano described how all the rooms are same-sided—organized in such a way that equipment and supplies are always located in the same place—"a nurse can literally put out his or her hand and find the supplies and equipment needed." The flows and zones for caregivers, patients, and families are clear and built into the designs, eliminating the need for hunting and gathering. Nurses can focus on the kind of work they should be doing: assessment and patient interactions.

Caregivers are organized into multidisciplinary teams, with physicians, nurses, dieticians, social workers, the palliative team, pastoral workers, and therapists readily available on the unit. As a result, nurses do not have to do time-consuming coordination work and can focus on care. Even the quality and outcome research staff are located on the unit, not in an administrative building. "System connections are everywhere," Bisognano said. "Patients are getting better care . . . in the hospital, prehospital, and also in the community for hospice."

Technology is used to support the frontline staff, with physicians and nurses collaborating on the design and use of technology. For example, technology links the staff remotely for direct patient visual and vital-sign monitoring. Because of these technology-mediated connections, "the sense of trust in the nursing staff is palpable."

The nursing staff returns and earns that trust. For example, when a flood in Cedar Rapids forced 300 patients to be evacuated from the hospital within 3 hours, many off-duty nurses arrived to move sandbags and transport those patients to other hospitals as far as 200 miles away.

Bisognano offered six priorities for the committee to consider. "If each of these changes happened in hospitals across the United States, quality and safety would be increased and costs would be reduced," she explained.

1. *Redesign care to optimize nurses' professional expertise and knowledge.* The goal should be for nurses to spend 60 percent of their time in direct patient care (RWJF and IHI, 2007). According to Bisognano, when this goal is met, not only will nurses be happier in their work, but also they will be providing care that is more effective and less costly. "Increasing value not only produces better efficiency, but also produces better outcomes."

2. *Focus on transformational leadership at all levels.* Nurses should be engaged and empowered to act as leaders at every level, Bisognano said. For example, nurses should be on hospital boards to think strategically about change—"How do we get nursing to help patients across the vast continuum of care?" Nurse leaders should work side by side with physicians to design the quality priorities for the organization. "All frontline nurses deserve training in quality improvement so they can redesign the processes of care at a patient's bedside."

3. *Work together to ensure safe and reliable care in acute settings.* Today, few hospitals have effectively implemented systems to identify and reduce errors. Yet the safety literature suggests that more than 70 percent of errors happen not because of incompetence, but because of system failures (Leape et al., 1993). Each failure should be used as a lesson to make system improvements. Examples of learning systems include medication system redesign, end-of-life best practices, and the use of rapid-response teams to rescue patients when their condition deteriorates.

4. *Build systems and cultures that encourage, support, and spread vitality and teamwork in all areas of nursing.* Bisognano said she has seen nurses walk off the unit at the end of the day exhausted from working in poorly designed workflow processes, and without the skills they need to make the changes on the front line. She also has seen nurses who feel fulfilled and vital, and who are respected at the end of a long and hard shift because work processes have been designed to support their professional skills. For example, health professionals who are confident in their ability to communicate with coworkers about concerns produce better patient outcomes and are more satisfied and engaged in their work (Maxfield et al., 2005).

5. *Put structures and processes into place that ensure patient-centered care.* Such care honors the whole person and family, respects individual values and choices, and ensures continuity of care as patients transfer from one setting to another. In most hospitals, systems and processes are still designed to meet the needs of the providers, not the patients. In Bisognano's experience, care teams that work with patients and families to establish daily goals and patient preferences not only provide better care, but result in fewer readmissions, failures, and complications. Nurses are the logical people to create innovative new models to spread the best clinical care across the continuum.

6. *Create a national learning system to make all models and prototypes accessible to nurses at all levels everywhere in the country.* Bisognano repeated Marilyn Chow's injunction: "We are excellent at everything, but excellence is just not everywhere." The tools exist to close gaps and fulfill the promise to patients.

VALUE, RELIABILITY, AND COLLABORATION IN NURSING

Tamra Minnier, chief quality officer at the University of Pittsburgh Medical Center (UPMC), emphasized three points that would make a great impact in the future of nursing:

1. The courage to stop doing work that is not value added.
2. The ability to build reliable nursing care delivery systems.
3. The redesign of care teams led by nurses.

As a simple example of work that is not value added, Minnier cited fall risk assessments. At UPMC, the fall screening admission assessment had grown to 24 sections on paper and 30 sections as an electronic record. A major redesign effort reduced the size of the form to just three questions. "The third question really threw people—in your judgment, as a nurse, do you think this patient is going to fall? God forbid that we let you think!" The redesign led to a 90 percent reduction in nurses' time to fill out the electronic record and an 87 percent reduction in the time to fill out the paper record.

Although the design seems straightforward, said Minnier, it actually required considerable courage. People had a tendency to ask, "What about this or what about that?" But building systems to the exception rather than the rule makes them cumbersome and difficult to successfully manage.

Reliability is a design feature well known to engineers, but rarely emphasized in nursing. The example Minnier used to describe the importance of reliability is the failure to prevent skin breakdowns. Nearly 500 patients at UPMC hospitals develop hospital-acquired pressure ulcers over the course of a year. Nurses "feel absolute personal failure when that happens." A major cause for the problem is that nurses too often have to combine work that needs to be done reliably with work that arises unpredictably. "We expect people to do steady, consistent work while they are being interrupted hundreds and hundreds of times a day."

Reliability needs to be a bedrock feature of nursing systems, Minnier said. Reliable work is the essential, routine work done to maintain basic patient care standards. It includes tasks such as admission assessments, medication distribution, assistance with activities of daily living, turning, risk assessment, wandering assessment, comfort rounds, and environmental checks. Unreliable, or unpredictable, work occurs randomly over the course of 24 hours and includes activities such as preparing or transferring a patient for testing or procedures, answering call bells, family communication, placing a patient in isolation, and emergencies. Splitting of routine and unexpected tasks will allow reliability to be built back into the systems and will allow teams to be built around these different sets of responsibilities.

Finally, nurses need to lead care teams. In the past, physicians have often been seen as the "captain of the ship" in hospitals. "We need our physician colleagues for many components of care delivery, but we know, in the end, who actually delivers that care and coordinates that care: It is the nurse," Minnier said. Nursing staff need the right tools and nurse-driven protocols to redesign nursing and transform care at the bedside. For example, teams might be designed that include a care nurse leader; a reliable, uninterrupted rounder doing predictable tasks; a medication nurse; and so on. "I don't have all the answers. None of us has the answers individually, but collectively we do." The important point is that a team is needed to care for a patient—and the patient should be seen as part of that team.

Patients deserve to have their needs met every time, Minnier said, and staff deserve to do an excellent job every time. The system needs to support both these needs by making work easier. Redesign of the system needs to build reliability into processes, promote continuous workflow by reducing interruptions, assign tasks to the right individuals, remove waste and redundancy, and test in order to learn. "It begins with trust— trusting what we know is right."

Nursing has arrived at the right moment to make changes, Minnier said. "We have been in this current state for way too long," she said. "It has a degree of inertia. It sometimes feels insurmountable. . . . But we must muster the courage to make it different."

REACTIONS FROM RESPONDER PANEL

In response to the presentations from Bisognano and Minnier, Dr. Julia Hallisy, a dentist representing the Empowered Patient Coalition, observed that patients and their families are "the most underused resources in the acute care system today." Patients recognize that nurses need to be as efficient and as productive as possible, and many patients are willing and able to be engaged as care partners. Patients know they will be safer when nurses spend more time at the bedside. They also know that, when a new procedure or technology is implemented at a hospital, nurses are usually the ones who will be doing the implementation and will be the first to know what works and what does not work. Patients and their families realize that the person at the bedside is the one who first recognizes the signs of deterioration, but this requires that nurses spend time at the bedside rather than being constantly distracted. Finally, patients and their families value communication with physicians and nurses, requiring that patients and their families be encouraged to communicate, educated in the best ways to communicate, and included on formal bodies such as advisory committees so their voices can be heard.

Dr. Joseph Guglielmo, professor and chair of the Department of Clinical Pharmacy at the University of California–San Francisco School of Pharmacy, emphasized that communication has to occur among the staff in a hospital, including between pharmaceutical services and nursing. Sometimes this relationship can be adversarial, but his institution has fostered a collaboration that is based on being proactive rather than reactive. "We cannot communicate too much, and I include my hospitalist colleagues and other physicians in those problem-solving processes as well," Guglielmo said.

Dr. Kurt Swartout, chief of Hospital Medicine at Kaiser Permanente Roseville Medical Center, pointed out that quality measures are often based on single outcomes, such as falls or infections. However, emphasizing those measures risks missing the overall picture. Many patients present with so many different problems that outcome-based measures would be a better way to drive quality improvements, he said.

Dr. Bernice Coleman, acute care nurse practitioner at Cedars-Sinai Medical Center, said nurses have the answers to many problems if they are given the opportunity to develop those answers. "To have nurses bring value to some of the solutions, we, as leaders, have to allow that to happen." At the same time, leaders must act from a patient-centered perspective. Once patients are discharged back into the community, care providers need to stay connected with the patient. "We [need to] design systems such that the continuing care that happens in the hospital, with nurses and teams, continues after discharge."

Finally, Nancy Chiang, former secretary/treasurer of the California Student Nurses Association, noted that student nurses often believe they do not get to spend enough time with nurses in a clinical setting learning their profession. Improvements in communications between patients and nurses also would be beneficial for nurses and nursing students. Similarly, students could benefit by spending more time with other members of care teams.

COMMITTEE QUESTION-AND-ANSWER SESSION

In response to a question about how patient-centered care should be defined, Bisognano said patients should be asked to rate their agreement with the following statement: *They give me all the care I want and need, exactly when and where I want and need it.* She agreed that many existing metrics looked at clinical processes rather than care from the perspective of the patient. She also noted that care is much more patient centered in other countries than in the United States. She described a friend's account of her father's experience after breaking a hip in England. "The day before he went home, a nurse-led squad arrived at the house . . . and went through the entire house with her mother. They installed a grab bar in the shower, a [seat] on the toilet so he could get up and down. They handed the mother the pain medication and went over diet. They tacked down the rugs and talked about how to take care of his wound. That is patient-centered care, and the patient won't be readmitted because the nurses are carrying that patient care from one setting to another. We need to figure out how to measure that."

Bisognano also pointed out that the involvement of students with nurses who have a variety of experiences and expertise is essential. She described a chief executive officer who posted a sign at his hospital saying, "Every patient deserves an experienced nurse, and every nurse deserves an experienced nurse." A metric such as years of experience among the nurses working per shift could help ensure that patients and other nurses benefit from experienced nurses.

In response to a question about how hospitals can use patients and their families as a resource, Minnier observed that patients and families can make a big difference in health care. For example, they can be given a specific assignment, such as keeping the head of a bed elevated to avoid ventilator-associated pneumonias. Her hospital also has implemented a program in which patients and families can call for rapid-response teams in case deterioration in a patient's condition is noted, providing "a set of eyes and ears that we don't have."

Minnier also provided several examples of nurse-specific protocols response to a question from the committee. She highlighted protocols such as deciding when to culture a patient for *Clostridium difficile* or knowing when a patient is ready to be discharged. "These levels of empowerment are some of the strategies for the future that we need to consider."

A questioner asked whether the current national discussion about health care reform might affect nursing. Bisognano replied that the national discussion has so far centered on health payment reform rather than health care reform. The IHI recently brought together representatives of 10 institutions that had low costs and high-quality outcomes at a meeting entitled "How Do They Do That?" These models of excellence need to become visible, she said, so that as health care reform progresses, any hospital can adapt proven practices to local circumstances.

Chow observed that a problem with health care is that "we all seem to learn the same thing over and over again." An infrastructure needs to be established that will allow the system to reach a higher level. How can high standards and best practices not only be identified, but disseminated and implemented?

A committee member asked what has kept the health care system from implementing efficient processes. Is it a lack of financial incentives, money, nurse empowerment, or some other factor? Chow replied that hospitals were not designed through a holistic process. Instead, departments created their own processes over many years, and these processes were not necessarily designed to work together or accommodate the needs of nurses and patients. Also, there is an inertia in hospitals that works against change and a "not invented here" syndrome that keeps promising innovations from other places from being accepted. Until departments come together to redesign care around the needs of patients, hospitals will continue to develop in a haphazard way.

Minnier noted that many leaders in hospitals do not fully understand the issues that face nursing and fail to keep the care of patients front and center, "whether [because of] unaligned incentives, lack of knowledge, or lack of understanding." National programs such as Transforming Care at the Bedside can elevate issues to a level beyond the institution and lead to meaningful change. Also, one step the IHI has taken is a program to build the skills of physicians, nurses, students, administrators, and others to fix broken processes on the front line.

4

Technology

TECHNOLOGY-ENABLED INNOVATION

The introduction of new technologies into hospitals is not an unfettered good, said Steven DeMello, research program director at the Public Health Institute. "If you can't identify ways in which you can improve practice, improve process, or improve business models, it does not have great value."

DeMello focused on what he called technology-enabled innovation—changes in practices, procedures, or business models that have technology at their heart. He also proposed a high standard for new technologies. He asserted that their adoption should lead to transformative practice that simultaneously improves clinical quality and reduces costs at a scale that can drive value across large sections of practice and large sections of the country.

As shown in Table 4-1, five areas of technology are especially promising:

1. Technologies related to ergonomics are very valuable and often overlooked. The combination of physically demanding work, an increasingly elderly and obese patient population, and an aging workforce is already producing high rates of work-related injuries. Patient lifting and transportation technologies, along with continued reductions in the size of diagnostic and therapeutic equipment, are unheralded but valuable advances that can be applied to nursing.

TABLE 4-1 Areas of Promising Technology Innovation

Area	Issues	Technologies
Ergonomics	Staff and patient safety	Patient lifts, mobile D&T equipment
Education and training	Recruitment and retention	E-learning, distance learning, simulation
Productivity	Communications and process streamlining	POCT, wireless, RTLS, facility design
Efficiency	Use of scarce, highly trained staff	Telemedicine, remote monitoring, care management
Clinical practice	New models of care	A-ICU,[a] family care units

[a]Ambulatory Intensive-Caring Units (A-ICU) is a model of primary care developed by Arnie Milstein. "The model pairs high-performing clinical teams with high-risk patients—those with chronic illnesses or socioeconomic issues that contribute to high healthcare usage. The aim is to prevent higher 'downstream' costs related to traditional primary care, specialty care and hospital admissions, by implementing these cost-saving features" (Shaw, 2009).

NOTES: A-ICU = Ambulatory Intensive-Caring Units; D&T = Diagnosis and Treatment; POCT = Point-of-Care Testing; RTLS = Real-Time Location Systems.

2. Education and training technologies such as e-learning, distance learning, and simulation can provide better and more flexible opportunities for nurses and nursing students across the country to learn from nursing professionals—an especially important consideration given projected shortages of direct caregivers.

3. Technologies that can improve nursing productivity include innovations related to better communications, streamlined processes, and improved coordination among caregivers at all levels. Foundational innovations include point-of-care testing, wireless communications, real-time location systems, and software that incorporates workflow data into facilities design. Individually and collectively, these innovations can increase nursing time at the bedside while reducing repetitive communications and administrative burdens. In particular, improvements in wireless communications and real-time location systems hold great promise in the next 2 to 5 years.

4. Technologies that can improve nursing efficiency can make the best possible use of increasingly scarce human resources. Foundational technologies include telemedicine, remote physiological and environmental monitoring, and care management. For example, telemedicine could support networks of care sites that are managed by highly skilled nurses. Such technologies also could provide much greater levels of care in homes and non-acute settings, which would have the additional benefit of reducing the workload at acute care sites.

5. Technologies that can change basic models of practice could result in much higher levels of bedside time and care management and decrease the burden of administration, communication, and documentation. For example, models of care could draw more heavily on other licensed and unlicensed caregivers, including family and friends, working under the direction of nursing care managers. Four specific technologies hold promise in the short term to help transform nursing through changes in practice models: point-of-care testing, wireless communications, real-time location systems, and telemedicine. The development of these technologies is accelerating, and current capabilities will grow rapidly in the next few years.

DeMello commented on the absence of electronic health records (EHRs) from this list of promising technologies. He said that EHRs are a foundational technology, but they are important to a much wider segment of the health care system than just nursing. In addition, EHRs should be seen as a floor, but not a ceiling; they are a base on which to build, but not the sole or even primary technological answer to improving care processes. He also expressed concern that the current focus on EHRs might have the unintended consequence of limiting the ability of caregivers and institutions to experiment with other technologies that could be extremely beneficial with or without an EHR.

A painful lesson learned from past experiences is that the "what" of technology adoption often obscures the "how." Specifically, how are technologies diffused within and across organizations? Diffusion depends not just on the technology, but on the regulatory and legal environment and on the investment that institutions make in diffusion. Laws and regulations related to scope of practice, supervision, and other aspects of care can slow or halt the diffusion of technologies that influence roles, supervision, or communication. Inconsistent policies across states can make it difficult to know what is legal in each jurisdiction and can obviate the benefits to natural markets that span legal boundaries.

Additionally, institutions often do not devote enough attention and resources to technology diffusion. "As an industry, we have gotten very skilled at trials, we are pretty spotty at initial implementation, and we are positively terrible at taking that implementation and replicating it consistently and appropriately across organizations," DeMello said. As the health care industry simultaneously consolidates and becomes more complex, it will be important to have broad-based, consistent application of technologies to catalyze the transformation of nursing.

TECHNOLOGY-ENABLED NURSING

Nurses have been using time-saving and lifesaving technologies for years, said Dr. Pamela Cipriano, former chief nursing officer at the University of Virginia Medical Center. In the 1970s, for example, nurses began to use technologies to monitor multiple critical care patients simultaneously, "so nurses were exposed to technology very early on in terms of looking at the explosion of the use of electronics in the patient care setting." But nurses have usually been passive consumers rather than active designers of technology. Rarely have they been involved in the design, testing, or purchasing of equipment. Cipriano recalled working in a cardiothoracic and trauma intensive care unit when a patient arrived from open-heart surgery with a brand new balloon pump in tow that none of the nurses had seen before. "There was no manual, no technical expert from the company. It is my hope that that doesn't happen anymore, although every once in a while we hear a horror story, which is why current regulations provide safeguards to prevent that," she said. "Today nurses also ensure proper use by being engaged in selection and implementation of patient care technologies."

By bringing value to nurses and patients, technology can save money, time, and lives. It can augment the delivery of nursing care, preserve the health of nurses, reduce unnecessary tasks, make it simpler and easier for nurses to conduct their daily activities, and reduce the potential for errors.

One crucial benefit technology can provide is a single set of clinical data. "Right now we have multiple professionals and providers collecting data that get hidden away in a variety of places, and some electronic records are difficult to navigate." As with the fragmented health care system, the result is fragmented documentation within electronic records, which multiplies the challenges of bringing all the information together to care for patients.

By involving nurses in the design—and not just the use—of technology, new devices and systems can be integrated so that they are as easy to use as possible. Nurses are eager to see the functionality that exists in consumer technologies being built into point-of-care technologies. They should be voice activated, handheld, and portable, and they should use biometrics and offer translation, Cipriano said.

Introducing equipment for equipment's sake does not help the nurse. Equipment needs to add value and efficiency to nursing rather than forcing nurses to also nurse the equipment. The nursing workflow is complex, which poses challenges to the adoption of technology. Nurses have a tendency to skip steps and are very good at jumping ahead to the next task that needs to be done. They quickly figure out how to cut corners. Some do not have the computer skills that would be ideal in today's nursing environment. If technologies are nurse-friendly, they can create safer, higher quality, and more efficient work environments and add value to the way that nurses coordinate and provide care. Greater nurse satisfaction leads to greater patient satisfaction.

Changing the nursing workflow first is more important, Cipriano said, than introducing a technology and hoping that it will change the workflow. One way to embed new workflows into technology is to build evidence-based and best practices into information systems. For example, systems can prioritize messages about patient conditions and feed that information to nurses and other caregivers in handheld devices so they can respond quickly to changing clinical conditions. Yet technologies also can be misused. For example, beds that vibrate do not mean that patients do not need to be turned.

Nurses still do a considerable amount of transcription. "If we know that the nurse is writing down data like vital signs and then putting them into a system later, it is incredibly inefficient. There are wireless devices that not only collect the vital signs, but transmit and embed those data into the information system. This fundamentally needs to be everywhere, not just in the places that have chosen to purchase that equipment."

The recent Technology Drill Down study done by the American Academy of Nursing has examined a variety of workflow issues, including medication administration, communication, timely acquisition and tracking of equipment and supplies, wireless monitoring, electronic clinical documentation, and patient identification, that could reduce error rates to zero. As a specific case, Cipriano observed that wireless patient monitoring "is finally taking off." Companies are doing the necessary work so that technologies integrated into a bed or mattress pad can monitor weight, blood pressure, heart rate, respiratory rate, or body movement. Such technologies also can be integrated into call or other communication system to alert nurses of patient changes. Another example of a smart system is a hospital bed that includes a translation feature so that routine questions can be asked in different languages. "Nurses have told us repeatedly that having translation at the point of care is becoming more and more critical."

The Drill Down study also looked at the desired outcomes of technology development and adoption. The most important were to reduce duplicative work, provide rapid access to other providers and resources, accomplish regulatory work, and improve the physical environment.

Cipriano made four specific suggestions regarding technology:

1. Include nursing workflow as a focus of health care information technology funding to ensure that systems and devices will enable nurses to be more efficient and produce safer care.
2. Advocate for nurses to be included in technology design and evaluation to enhance rapid adoption.
3. Ensure that nurses are seen as meaningful users of technology.
4. Support nurses in moving high-technology care into the hospital setting of the future—the home and community.

Adopting these suggestions would "make sure that we are, in fact, transforming the way that we deliver care and are using technology as an adjunct to do that," Cipriano said.

REACTIONS AND QUESTIONS

Joseph Guglielmo asked why promising new models for nursing have not moved forward in many cases. He speculated that one reason is a lack of evidence about their effectiveness. The assumption is that new systems and technologies have undergone a quality assurance program, but that is not necessarily the case. "My take-home [message] is that we need more evidence, we need not to be afraid to ask questions, to say, 'What is the true value?'" Furthermore, these assessments need to consider the workflow of all care providers, including nurses.

Today's patients know and like technology, said Julia Hallisy. Patients realize that technology can improve their safety, help keep nurses at their bedside, and improve communication among the members of their care teams. Patients and families can be frustrated when a caregiver is not aware of a changed treatment plan or new order. Patients know that such communication failures can be avoided through something as easy as a wireless phone. The result for nurses is that patients and family members can become agitated, which places a burden on nurses. "Patients are going to expect it and they are going to demand it," she said.

In response to a question about the use of technology to provide real-time access and greater patient involvement, which was referred to by the questioner as more patient-controlled care, Kurt Swartout recounted his experiences with an electronic medical record system used in his hospital for the past 14 months. He brings a computer to the patient's bedside so they can review test results and other information together. In addition, specialists on a care team can instantly have information about a patient and provide immediate input to decisions. "I don't think we realized how valuable it is to have information . . . that everyone can look at," he noted. The system also allows caregivers to gain information from nurses, "so it has increased the sophistication of our conversation."

One challenge, Swartout continued, is to reduce the time spent on documentation while improving its quality; nurses spend about 35 percent of their time on documentation. One way to do so is through auto-correct options that reduce the amount of typing needed. Voice recognition technology also can allow caregivers to dictate information to a computer without having to type that information.

A viewer of the webcast of the forum wrote to point out that technology can not only collect patient data, but assist with the analysis and review of that data. DeMello agreed and extended the argument to technologies that are less clinical in nature, but still can improve health care. An example is a set of databases that track which caregivers are associated with which patients. A roadblock to the implementation of such technologies, he said, is managing the data behind the scenes that the technology generates. "We are much less far along in managing the complexity than we [should be]."

Caregivers and health care institutions also need to be willing to use technology to interact with patients and families, Cipriano said. This should be a point of emphasis in education and training, so that future professionals are ready from the beginning of their careers to use technologies at the point of care.

In response to a question about whether some technologies have detrimental rather than beneficial effects, Guglielmo agreed that many technologies have unintended consequences. Indeed, all technologies have such consequences, but they are not well studied scientifically. DeMello divided such consequences into two categories: technologies that do active harm or are not consistent with good care, and technologies that deliver minuscule benefits for massive investments. The latter case is even more important, more difficult to solve, and harder to reverse, he said. Cipriano observed that positive and negative consequences of new technologies are part of the adoption curve of any technology. "It reinforces the fact that we do need to look at and measure the impact of technology so that we can make the right decisions and take it away if necessary," Cipriano said.

In response to a question about how technology could be used to shift acute care out of hospitals or keep patients from having to come to hospitals, Marilyn Chow discussed technologies that enable the "hospital at home." In addition, Bernice Coleman described ways in which technology can improve continuity of care. For example, in transitioning from a hospital to the community, care inside the hospital could be linked to virtual care outside the hospital. Not just patients and their families, but entire communities could be supported in the use of health care technologies. Nurses could be at the center of this transition, but they need to have access to information, technology, and support to fill this role.

Cipriano also pointed to telehealth technologies that patients and families can use to manage chronic conditions that in the past would have required being in a hospital. For example, technologies such as cell phones can help teens to manage diabetes or nutritional choices. "There are nurse-led programs around the country that are making a difference in being able to inform consumers at any age and allow them to participate in the management of their health care," Cipriano said.

Similarly, the Veterans Administration (VA) has been working on the home management of chronic diseases with "terrific results," DeMello said. The VA "spent a considerable amount of time figuring out the logistics—how they could use multiple units, how they could make sure people in the home were supported, how the education happens. It is an interesting blueprint for what's possible."

A final comment from a webcast observer noted that technology only works as well as the person using it. If a health care organization does not maintain a technology, or a nurse distrusts it, a technology will not be effective.

5

Interdisciplinary Collaboration

FOSTERING COLLABORATION AMONG HEALTH CARE PROFESSIONALS

Studies of the context in which health care is delivered date back at least to the reforms instituted by Florence Nightingale in the 1850s, said Dr. Pamela Mitchell, professor of Biobehavioral Nursing and Health Systems at the University of Washington and president of the American Academy of Nursing. Since then, many other studies have looked at issues such as continuous quality improvement, patient safety, and crew resource management as ways to improve interprofessional collaboration.

In a demonstration project conducted in the 1980s by the American Association of Critical-Care Nurses, a positive work environment characterized by interprofessional collaboration and a high level of expertise on the part of both nurses and physicians had lower-than-expected mortality and very high patient satisfaction (Mitchell et al., 1989). As this association was tested in a larger number of critical care units with generally good mortality outcomes, an association between positive work environments and reduced mortality proved to be elusive. Nevertheless, this study, and several others conducted over the years, showed that a positive work environment led to greater retention of registered nurses (RNs) because they developed a sense of having a greater influence over the working environment, more collaboration with physicians and other health care workers, and access to a wider variety of conflict resolution skills. These studies also showed that physicians had better perceptions of the quality of nurses, other physicians, and the unit as a whole, while RNs had better perceptions of overall quality and patient satisfaction

(Ingersoll and Schmitt, 2004; Mitchell et al., 1996). Together, this research contributed to a recommendation made in 2003 at a summit sponsored by the Institute of Medicine that health professions education should focus on core competencies for all health professionals so they can work in interdisciplinary teams, use evidence-based practice, provide patient-centered care, apply quality improvement principles, and use information technologies, as shown in Figure 5-1 (IOM, 2003).

Since World War II numerous attempts have been made to create educational endeavors that bring people together across professions. For example, the rehabilitation of soldiers wounded in World War II required the input of many people in both acute care and rehabilitation. The Great Society of the 1960s brought a resurgence of these educational efforts, augmented by the increased use of technology in intensive care units. In the mid-1970s and 1980s, there was dedicated federal and private funding for interdisciplinary education (Baldwin, 1996). Periods of health care reform tend to produce greater funding for such endeavors, Mitchell said, which means that interprofessional education could again receive greater attention in the years ahead.

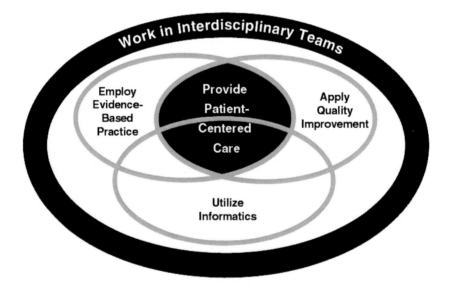

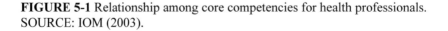

FIGURE 5-1 Relationship among core competencies for health professionals. SOURCE: IOM (2003).

In recent years, the University of Washington and many other educational institutions have experimented with different forms of interprofessional education. These approaches were grounded in the belief that collaboration requires understanding and respect for others' expertise as well as competence in one's own practice discipline. Collaboration also requires understanding the context and complexity of the health of a population, which requires basic group skills such as conflict resolution (Mitchell et al., 2006). However, these approaches to interprofessional collaboration initially underplayed the importance of including the patient, family, and others in the community as part of the care team, Mitchell said. "That is something that I believe needs to be emphasized as we move forward."

Several years ago, Mitchell served on an IOM committee that produced the report *Keeping Patients Safe: Transforming the Work Environment of Nurses* (IOM, 2004). The report recommended that hospitals and educational institutions support nursing staff in ongoing acquisition and maintenance of knowledge and skills. It also recommended adopting mechanisms such as interdisciplinary rounds and ongoing education in interdisciplinary collaboration.

Work from Dr. Stephen Shortell and colleagues about successful quality improvement programs forms a useful framework for identifying the components of successful interprofessional education programs (Shortell et al., 1996). Strategically, such programs need institutional leadership and faculty champions. Structurally, they need consistent institutional policies and a physical infrastructure. Technical knowledge and skills need to be combined with a meaningful focus. In addition, a culture of collaboration, strong personal relationships, and time and flexibility are needed to make programs work.

Mitchell offered a single recommendation: Academic institutions and health care organizations need to make a real commitment to interprofessional education that develops and sustains collaborative skills, both before and after licensure. The recommendation is not new, Mitchell said. "But let's make it real this time. . . . That means committing money, committing resources, and committing structure."

DISRUPTIVE BEHAVIOR, NURSING CARE,
AND PATIENT SAFETY

In 2000, Dr. Alan Rosenstein, vice president and medical director for VHA West Coast, began to study the effects of disruptive behavior on nursing care and patient safety. Rosenstein defined disruptive behavior as "any inappropriate behavior, confrontation, or conflict ranging from verbal abuse to physical or sexual harassment." Disruptive behavior in the workplace is a serious concern for those who experience it and witness it, as well as for the patients being cared for in this negative environment. As demonstrated in Figure 5-2, there is relatively little physical abuse, Rosenstein said, but there is "a lot of yelling, a lot of screaming, a lot of condescending, berating behavior, particularly in front of peers."

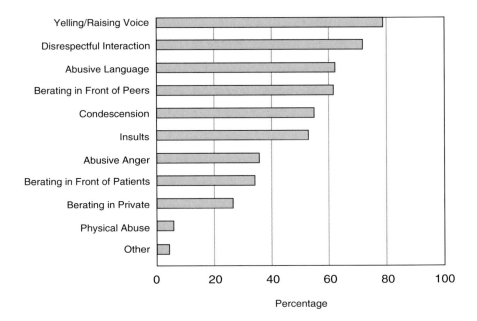

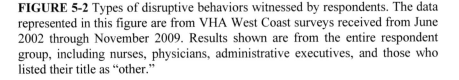

FIGURE 5-2 Types of disruptive behaviors witnessed by respondents. The data represented in this figure are from VHA West Coast surveys received from June 2002 through November 2009. Results shown are from the entire respondent group, including nurses, physicians, administrative executives, and those who listed their title as "other."

Little if any research had been published on the subject of disruptive behavior before, but an initial survey opened up a "Pandora's box," Rosenstein noted. The survey found a high incidence of disruptive behaviors among physicians, with a significant impact on nurse satisfaction and retention (Rosenstein, 2002; Rosenstein et al., 2002). A follow-up survey published in 2005 found that disruptive behavior by both physicians and nurses had a significant impact on clinical outcomes of care (Rosenstein and O'Daniel, 2005). Additional surveys in 2007 and 2008 documented a significant impact of disruptive behavior on clinical outcomes in high-stress areas such as surgery and cardiovascular specialties and on psychological factors (Rosenstein and O'Daniel, 2006, 2008a, 2008b). "Disruptive behavior has tremendous ramifications . . . and the data are striking," Rosenstein said.

According to these surveys, 77 percent of hospital personnel have witnessed disruptive behavior from a physician at their hospital and 65 percent have witnessed disruptive behavior from a nurse. Those figures rise to 88 and 73 percent, respectively, for surveys of RNs. Such behavior from physicians tends to be more overt, while among nurses it can be more subtle, "which is probably more disruptive because you don't know where you are at." Rosenstein's research also found that 60 to 70 percent of the adverse events that happen to patients can be traced to problems with communication. Furthermore, 50 percent of physicians are not good communicators, Rosenstein said.

The problem is not new, but bureaucracy, hierarchies, and politics have stymied efforts to deal with it, Rosenstein said. More recently, the effects of disruptive behavior on nurse and patient satisfaction and patient safety have increased focus on the problem. Surveys show that one third of nurses who leave hospitals do so at least in part because of disruptive physicians, which has become a particular concern as nursing shortages have become more pressing. Surveys also show that this disruptive behavior often leads to stress, frustration, loss of concentration, reduced collaboration, reduced information transfer, reduced communication, and impaired nurse–physician relationships.

Furthermore, surveys done by Rosenstein and his collaborators document a link between disruptive behavior and undesirable clinical outcomes, including adverse events, errors, increased mortality, and decreased patient safety, quality of care, and patient satisfaction, as shown in Figure 5-3. Among all personnel surveyed, 18 percent were aware of specific adverse effects that occurred as a result of disruptive behavior.

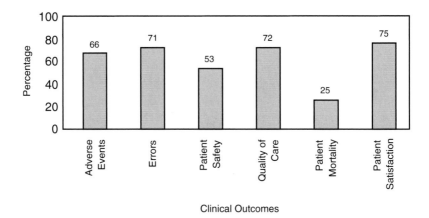

FIGURE 5-3 Linkage of disruptive behavior to undesirable clinical outcomes reported as occurring sometimes, frequently, or constantly. The data represented in this figure are from VHA West Coast surveys received from June 2002 through November 2009. As in Figure 5-2, results shown are from the entire respondent group, including nurses, physicians, administrative executives, and those who listed their title as "other."

Comments from individuals substantiated this finding, Rosenstein said. As one respondent wrote, "Most nurses are afraid to call Dr. X when they need to, and frequently won't call. Their patients' medical safety is always in jeopardy because of this." Another wrote, "Staff nurses advocated for better patient care, but M.D. [was] not willing to listen to reason. As a result the patient died. The doctor chose to undo all the help that various staff had been working on for weeks to get this patient the help so badly needed."

Many factors cause people to act and react the way they do in these situations, including age differences, gender, culture, ethnicity, values, experiences, training, and personality styles. Stress, frustration, fatigue, depression, substance abuse, or a lack of emotional intelligence can all contribute to the problem, as can situational factors such as the environment or the mood of the day.

Modifying behaviors can be difficult, but several steps could reduce disruptive behaviors. Organizations need to be committed to changing the culture, with endorsement from leadership. One way to approach the problem is with an internal survey, because staff typically do not want to discuss these issues in public. Education needs to occur across the board, from the senior level to students, including administrators and support staff. Advanced training can focus on the areas of diversity, competence (in both knowledge and communication), and assertiveness. Programs to reduce disruptive behavior need to offer structured training and educational programs, coaching support, endorsement by clinical champions, reinforcement of policies and procedures, a consistent process for reporting and follow-up for disruptive events, and strategies to enforce compliance through means such as intervention and feedback. Early intervention programs have the greatest chance of success (Rosenstein, 2009).

These steps need to be taken to reinforce patient safety initiatives, Rosenstein asserted. "What nurses really want is to feel that they are a part of the process, that they are respected, and that they have some participation in a patient's care plan."

REACTIONS AND QUESTIONS

Nancy Chiang remarked on the particular value of collaboration for students. "The willingness of the various disciplines in the hospital to work with students is crucial," she said. "Clinical time is very limited for us, so in addition to what we get from the nurses, what we get from the other specialties is just as important."

In response to a question about the best way for interprofessional education to occur, Mitchell cited a program at the University of Southampton in England in which teams of medical students, nurses, social workers, and pharmacists worked with particular units in the hospital to develop continuous quality improvement projects. Just being around people from other professions is not enough, she said. People need to work through problems together, often with the aid of a coach or facilitator.

In response to a question about whether an age and gender gap between physicians and nurses contributes to a lack of collaboration and whether narrowing that gap will change matters, Rosenstein responded that an "old guard" still exists in health care that has been doing business the same way for many years. "There are still enough of the old people around, and until we can convince them to make the right changes, it is going to be slow to happen."

Bernice Coleman agreed that bringing colleagues along in efforts to change the culture of health care can be difficult. She reiterated that all advanced-practice nurses should be part of an active interdisciplinary team during their training. "They are going to need to do that, and they are the clinical leaders, so I think it is a critical part of their education."

Finally, a viewer of the webcast commented that multidisciplinary education should include not just physicians and nurses, but hospital and health care administrators as well.

6

Summaries of Testimony

Prior to the forum in Los Angeles, a variety of stakeholders and the public were invited to submit written testimony to the committee in three areas of relevance to acute care: quality and safety, technology, and interdisciplinary collaboration. Those submitting written testimony were asked to describe innovative models in these three areas; barriers that nurses face in implementing these models; and how nurses could be further engaged or effectively used to advance quality and safety, technology, and interdisciplinary collaboration in acute care settings.

Nineteen people at the forum provided oral testimony for the Initiative on the Future of Nursing; in most cases, these individuals or the organizations they represented also presented written testimony. Many important ideas and suggestions for the initiative emerged from this testimony and are summarized below in the order in which the comments were made. This testimony should not be interpreted as positions or recommendations of the committee, the Robert Wood Johnson Foundation, or the Institute of Medicine.

Donna Herrin-Griffith, President
American Organization of Nurse Executives (AONE)

AONE has been working in a number of areas, said Herrin-Griffith, including identifying solutions for the shortage of nurses and faculty; addressing concerns about quality and safety; highlighting the importance of the environment in which care is provided; and emphasizing the need to transform care delivery to achieve the goals of safe, effective, patient-centered, timely, efficient, and equitable health care.

AONE has defined the key responsibilities for nurses in its *Guiding Principles for the Role of the Nurse in Future Patient Care Delivery*. The six elements of that model are the following:

1. The core of nursing is knowledge and caring.
2. Care is user based.
3. Knowledge for nursing is access based.
4. Knowledge for nursing is synthesized.
5. Care is provided through relationships, either in person or virtually.
6. The journey of care is managed through partnerships between patients and nurses.

Herrin-Griffith said these concepts embody a model of future care for the health care industry to develop and implement.

Nancy Donaldson, Co-Principal Investigator
Collaborative Alliance for Nursing Outcomes

A gap exists in efforts to engage hospitals in building capacity to reliably and strategically use measures to inform priorities and improve performance, said Donaldson. The Collaborative Alliance for Nursing Outcomes, which is the nation's oldest nursing quality database and a joint venture between the Association of California Nurse Leaders and the American Nurses Association/California, advocated the following priorities:

1. Systematically build the capacity of clinicians and clinical administrator leaders to be accountable for and to use nursing quality data to guide decisions and performance.
2. Strengthen clinician access to and capacity to use web-based information.
3. Institutionalize ergonomic assessment of the potential impacts of patient care quality and safety initiatives on the nurse workload prior to implementation.
4. Invest in new metrics that add value for clinical administrative leaders and public policy stakeholders.
5. Operationalize the expectation that nurses systematically evaluate their practice.

6. Institutionalize and align measures in research, education, and practice.

Phyllis Gallagher, Nurse Attorney
(presenting on behalf of Teri Mills, National Nursing Network Organization)

Gallagher said that the U.S. Congress should enact legislation to create an Office of the National Nurse. The National Nursing Network Organization believes that creating this position could improve health literacy, heighten the visibility of nursing on a national basis, promote the use of patients as caregivers to lower costs, and be a voice for national learning. The office could mobilize volunteers for projects such as adopting a school and school readiness programs.

Nearly 80 groups have already endorsed this proposal. "I would urge you to exercise your rights as citizens and try to promote this," said Gallagher.

Suzanne Boyle, Vice President for Patient Care Services
New York-Presbyterian Hospital/Weill Cornell

Boyle said the call for nurses to be transformational leaders is absolutely clear. As a result, an infrastructure is needed to identify best practices quickly and disseminate them, thus inspiring innovation. Also, Boyle indicated that examination of the roles of nurses must emphasize quality, safety, transitional models of care, and cross-disciplinary work.

Kathy Dawson, President
Association of California Nurse Leaders (ACNL)

To ensure that nurses provide competent, safe, and quality patient care in a complex health care environment, the current workforce must be retooled to elevate the standard of practice and to prepare the future workforce to meet the challenges of an ever-changing world, said Dawson. Knowledge is exploding in all facets of health care, and technology is changing the way nurses practice every day. To keep pace, the art and science of nursing must evolve.

Expecting that newly graduated registered nurses can perform immediately at the proficient level is inconsistent with the evidence of what is possible in the novice-to-expert model of practice development, Dawson said. The ACNL, in conjunction with other professional organizations in California, is developing transitional competencies based on the Quality and Safety Education for Nurses model as a framework for novice nurses in their first year of practice. These transitional competencies are meant to reinforce patient care practices that are safe and of high quality. In addition to the theoretical and didactic learning that takes place in nursing schools, the competencies learned from immersion in the role of the professional nurse are essential to gaining the experience nurses need. In particular, mandatory residencies are critical to prepare the registered nurse of the future, Dawson said.

Margaret Talley, Clinical Nurse Specialist
Palomar Pomerado Health
(presenting on behalf of Christine Filipovich, National Association of
Clinical Nurse Specialists)

The clinical nurse specialist (CNS) plays an essential role in acute care and in the future of nursing, said Talley. CNSs are leaders of interdisciplinary teams that improve the safety and quality of acute care by translating clinical expertise and integrating scientific knowledge and methods to design evidence-based solutions. They address the big picture in three key spheres of influence in acute care: the patients, nursing and the nursing staff, and the health care system as a whole.

CNSs' research and design solutions to the various problems and complications that arise in vulnerable patient populations, such as geriatric, pediatric oncology, neurology, psychology, rehabilitation, and emergency room populations. Programs developed by CNSs and implemented by interdisciplinary health care teams prevent avoidable complications, including patient falls, medication errors, hospital-acquired pressure ulcers, and infections. CNSs also act as faculty and mentors for new nurses and nurses pursuing advanced practice education.

The CNS is the ideal academic liaison for nursing schools to ensure a safe and comprehensive acute care learning experience, Talley said. Few other providers are prepared or in a position to design and implement the safety and quality solutions offer by CNSs.

DeAnn McEwen, Staff Nurse
Intensive Care Unit, Long Beach Memorial Medical Center
(presenting on behalf of Gerard Brogan, California Nurses Association)

The most critical barrier to the health, welfare, and safety of patients in acute care settings is the lack of unified, mandated safe staffing standards, including the lack of the right to advocate in most states in the exclusive interests of the patient without fear of retaliation, McEwen said.

Staffing standards are essential for the provision of competent, safe, and effective care. McEwen indicated that clearly defined, legally protected, and enforceable duties and rights for direct care registered nurses to advocate exclusively for the interest of patients are also needed, as well as whistleblower protections that encourage patients, registered nurses, and other health care personnel to notify government and private accreditation entities of suspected unsafe patient conditions.

According to McEwen, numerous studies done by the nation's most respected scientific and medical researchers affirm the significance to patient safety of direct care registered nurses-to-patient ratios. Improved staffing ratios have been associated with reductions in hospital-related mortality, in failures to rescue, and in lengths of stay, she said.

Hospitals are required to demonstrate they have mechanisms in place to collect and analyze patient outcome data with input from the nursing staff while incorporating clinical decision-making technologies. McEwen said human cognition is superior to machine intelligence, so there must be a strong commitment to preserve effective interdisciplinary collaborations.

The greatest barrier to interdisciplinary collaboration in acute care settings is access to entries made by other disciplines on the patient electronic record, McEwen said. Registered nurses have a unique patient advocacy role in the health care delivery system, and technology should be used to augment that role. In analyzing the safety, therapeutic value, and effectiveness of any technology, registered nurses must be able to explore the potential of technology to replace human interaction and to supplant critical thinking and independent clinical judgment with rigid clinical pathways. Health care providers must seek to control technology, not allow it to control health care.

Joyce Sensmeier, Cochair
Alliance for Nursing Informatics

Nurses play an important role in leveraging health information technology to improve patient safety, quality, and the efficiency of care delivery, Sensmeier said. They are also integral to achieving a vision to adopt and implement electronic health record (EHR) systems in a meaningful way. Sensmeier said that meaningful use of health information technology, when combined with best practice and evidence-based care, will improve health care for all Americans. The future of nursing relies on this transformation as well as on the important role of nurses in achieving a digital revolution.

Sensmeier indicated that nurses must be supported in a health care environment that adequately enables their knowledge-based work in a variety of roles. These roles include being leaders in the effective design and use of EHRs; integrators of information; full partners in decision making; care coordinators across disciplines; experts in improving quality, safety, and efficiency and in reducing health disparities; advocates for engaging patients and families; contributors to standardized EHR infrastructure; researchers on safe patient care; and educators for preparing the workforce.

Michelle Troseth, Chief Professional Practice Officer
Clinical Practice Model Resource Center/Elsevier

The CPM Consortium provides an infrastructure in which nurses and interdisciplinary partners can come together and create best places to give and receive care. Clinicians can focus on the fundamental elements that enable integration of quality care, technology, and interdisciplinary collaboration and make the combination come alive.

Troseth noted that the consortium has developed innovative, technology-leading, intentionally designed automation (IDA) at the point of care in partnership with multiple health information technology vendors. This system enables capture of the patient's story, development of an individualized evidence-based plan of care using clinical practice guidelines, assessments and interventions within the context of the patient's diagnosis and situation, and evaluation of progress toward goals.

The consortium has more than 125 acute care settings that have nurses and interdisciplinary teams using IDA within the CPM Framework. Outcome measures include reduced patient falls, reduced pressure ulcers, exceeding national and regional benchmarks by 85 to 95 percent, and increased nurse satisfaction, Troseth said. CPM Consortium sites also have been national exemplars for the TIGER (Technology and Informatics Guiding Education Reform) initiative, Sigma Theta Tau International, and American Nurses Credentialing Center Magnet-Designated Hospitals.

Dianne Moore, Vice President of Nursing Academics
West Coast University (presenting on behalf of Tina Johnson,
American College of Nurse Midwives)

Childbirth is the leading reason for admission to U.S. hospitals, and hospitalization is the most costly component of U.S. health care. Combined hospital charges for childbirth and care for newborns in 2004 were $75 billion, said Moore. This amount far exceeded that for any other condition, yet pregnancy is a normal, natural physiologic event.

Moore noted that various forces have led to a style of care that is ill suited to the great majority of mothers and babies who are healthy and have reason to expect an uncomplicated birth. For example, Childbirth Connection's national Listening to Mothers II survey found that professionals tried to induce labor 41 percent of the time; 32 percent of deliveries were cesarean-section deliveries; and 25 percent of births involved episiotomies. Due to the considerable overuse of these and other common interventions, many women experience risk without benefit, Moore said. Conversely, many beneficial practices with excellent safety profiles are underused.

Using the appropriate mix of providers and limiting the overuse of technology can provide desirable benefits, Moore indicated. For example, the Centering Health Care Institute, a nonprofit organization with offices in Cheshire, Connecticut, is seeking to change the paradigm of health services to a group care model to improve the overall health of mothers, babies, and new families across the life cycle. The Institute was incorporated in 2001, and there are now more than 300 sites led by nurse midwives across the United States that employ this group care model. Moore also cited research conducted by Yale University of more than 1,000 women in public clinics in New Haven, Connecticut, and Atlanta that demonstrated a 33 percent overall reduction in preterm births for women receiving this type of group care and a 40 percent reduction for the African American women in the same study group (Ickovics et al., 2007). In addition, Moore suggested that midwives should have their own independent admissions privileges.

Barbara Nichols, Chief Executive Officer
CGFNS (Commission on Graduates of Foreign Nursing Schools)
International

The mobility and migration of nurses worldwide and their impact on the global delivery of health services and nursing shortages have become topics of international debate. Although the recruitment of foreign-educated nurses traditionally has been perceived as an immediate and temporary solution to U.S. nursing shortages, foreign-educated nurses are already vital, essential, and permanent members of the U.S. nursing workforce, said Nichols. The majority of these nurses enter on occupational, spousal, or family visas that are permanent. Their skill mix and productivity are critical factors in the outcomes of health care delivery.

Accordingly, employers and institutions should make long-term investment in advanced education for faculty and leadership roles, Nichols indicated. CGFNS data suggest that the majority of foreign-educated nurses work in acute care settings, are an average of 15 years younger than their American counterparts, hold Baccalaureate degrees, bring 1 to 5 years of nursing experience to their positions, and are viewed as safe and competent practitioners. Yet these factors often are not considered in making short-term initial placement or long-term leadership decisions, she noted.

Foreign-educated nurses have been and will continue to be a vital part of the U.S. nursing workforce. Foreign-educated nurses represent an underused and valuable resource both within and outside of acute care settings, Nichols said.

Dana Alexander, Chief Nursing Officer
GE Healthcare

TIGER is a national collaborative of nurses from various sectors, including administration, practice, education, informatics, technology, organizations, government agencies, vendors, and more than 100 specialty nursing organizations. This collaboration is bridging the quality chasm with health information technology, enabling nurses to use informatics in practice and education to provide safer and higher quality care, Alexander said.

Alexander described three priorities from the TIGER collaborative:

1. Develop a nursing workforce that is capable of using EHRs to improve the delivery of health care.
2. Engage more nurses in leading both the development of a national health care information technology infrastructure and health care reform.
3. Accelerate adoption of smart, standards-based, interoperable technology that will make health care delivery safer, more efficient, timely, accessible, and patient centered while also reducing the burden on nurses.

Linda Arkava, Swedish Medical Center/First Hill (Seattle)
(presenting on behalf of Valerie Tate, Nurse Alliance of SEIU [Service Employees International Union] Healthcare)

The SEIU Healthcare Nurse Alliance advocates for quality improvement from the point of care by frontline nurses and other members of the health care team in partnership with hospital employers. Arkava said a true collaboration recognizes nurses' capacity to use their expert knowledge to solve problems and provides them with an equal role in defining and implementing a quality agenda. This requires committed leadership and equal accountability for shared goals from hospital executives, union leaders, organizations representing the nursing profession, and practicing nurses. Arkava indicated that frontline nurses should be engaged in the design, development, implementation, and evaluation of nursing innovations and solutions, whether for models of care or new technologies.

Frontline nurses also should be involved in the decisions and implementation of evidence-based policies, practices, and work environments for improved patient outcomes, increased nurse professional satisfaction, and increased safety for all, Arkava said. For example, Swedish Medical Center is using a collaborative model through unit-based staffing committees—which include nurses, ancillary staff, and managers—that are developing evidence-based staffing plans submitted with the units' yearly budget requests. Staffing effectiveness data will be collected to build adequate staffing and cultures of safety.

Improvements in patient outcomes, financial outcomes, and professional satisfaction exist where partnerships between SEIU nurses and employers have been built on shared priorities and responsibilities for quality, Arkava said. The most important and consistent feedback received from practicing nurses is that to provide quality and safe patient care, there needs to be not only standards for adequate staffing, but real oversight for compliance, Arkava noted.

Cathy Rick, Chief Nursing Officer
Department of Veterans Affairs

Acute care has become a fast-paced, episodic set of intensive events that requires system redesign to support the work of nursing. This system design needs not only to transform care at the bedside, but across the continuum of care, Rick said. Acute care nursing requires a cadre of nurses who are well prepared to provide focused attention to clinical surveillance and targeted, proven interventions that are coordinated with interdisciplinary care partners. She noted elements in moving toward not just a patient-centered, but also a patient-driven, model of care that includes the role of the clinical nurse leader (CNL), data-driven staffing methodologies, registered nurse residencies, and structured language for nursing documentation.

The CNL is an essential component of the patient care delivery model of the future, Rick said. CNLs are master clinicians who advance nursing practice at the point of care through application and dissemination of evidence-based nursing practice and system redesign. The CNL is prepared at a master's degree level as a generalist who is an expert in managing care challenges from a clinical perspective. Rick indicated that the Veterans Administration has fully endorsed this new nursing role and has a comprehensive plan to implement the role across all settings by the year 2016. Early findings demonstrate a positive impact on financial indicators, quality of care, and patient satisfaction.

Rick highlighted three areas to consider about the future of nursing:

1. Staffing methodologies, including workload and outcome indicators, need to be embedded in EHRs.

2. Funded and mandated registered nurse residencies are very important to consider.
3. To advance the understanding of nursing and nursing contributions, a standardized and structured language is needed that is embedded in the documentation system.

Penny Overgaard, Adult Cystic Fibrosis Program Coordinator
Phoenix Children's Hospital

Patient education is a critical element in the future of nursing. Patients are being discharged from acute care facilities sicker and earlier than ever before, and this trend will continue. As a result, patients and their families spend more time in self-care than they do in the care of a nurse, Overgaard said. Even something as simple as knowing who to call after discharge may be left undone in patient education. Much education is done in a hurry, is not completed, or is not understood when it is done, she explained.

Nurses are uniquely qualified to use their professional expertise to provide individualized education to patients. Nursing education at the college level and continuing education must emphasize how to assess learning readiness, ability, and literacy and provide an understanding of the impact of social disparities on patient education, said Overgaard.

Overgaard indicated that nursing research should explore the connection between patient education and positive outcomes so that people know there is value in having nurses teach. Finally, she said that future care models must value patient education, allow nurses time to teach in acute settings, and design novel ways to extend patient education into communities.

Elissa Brown, President
American Nurses Association of California

The involvement of nurses in new health care models and in designing and using technology needs to be supported, Brown said. In addition, mental health care, long-term care, hospice care, and palliative care have good models for interdisciplinary collaboration that need to be examined. She suggested using the term "health care home models" instead of "medical home models." Finally, Brown indicated that nurses need to be members of committees involved in decisions that affect patient care.

Carol Hartigan
American Association of Critical-Care Nurses

The American Association of Critical-Care Nurses considers acute and critical care to be on a continuum. Acutely ill patients are everywhere—from the intensive care unit to the home. Matching nurse competencies to patient needs is important, said Hartigan.

Beverly Malone, Chief Executive Officer
National League for Nursing

Health care teams need to include allied health colleagues such as licensed practical nurses and other care providers, particularly as medicine moves toward telemedicine and out of the hospital care, Malone said.

Kathy Harren, Chief Nurse Executive
Providence Little Company of Mary

The initiatives launched by the Institute for Healthcare Improvement have provided important lessons in the reform of care delivery, and the implementation of these models needs to be accelerated, Harren said. In addition, economic incentives will lead the transformation of the health care system and reveal the important and varied roles of nurses, both in the hospital and in other care delivery settings.

A

References

AHA (American Hospital Association). 2002. *It's in our hands: How hospital leaders can build a thriving workforce.* Chicago, IL: American Hospital Association.

Baldwin, D. 1996. Some historical notes on interdisciplinary and interprofessional education and practice in health care in the USA. *Journal of Interprofessional Care* 10(2):173-187.

Christensen, C. 1997. *The innovator's dilemma: When new technologies cause great firms to fail.* Cambridge, MA: Harvard Business School Press.

Christensen, C. 2009. *Key concepts—disruptive innovation.* http://www.claytonchristensen.com/disruptive_innovation.html (accessed December 16, 2009).

Hendrich, A., M. Chow, B. A. Skierczynski, and Z. Lu. 2008. A time and motion study: How do medical–surgical nurses spend their time? *The Permanente Journal* 12(3):37-46.

Ickovics, J. R., T. S. Kershaw, C. Westdahl, U. Magriples, Z. Massey, H. Reynolds, and S. S. Rising. 2007. Group prenatal care and perinatal outcomes: A randomized controlled trial. *Obstetrics and Gynecology* 110(2, Part 1):330-339.

Ingersoll, G., and M. Schmitt. 2004. Work groups and patient safety. In *Keeping patients safe: Transforming the work environment of nurses.* Washington, DC: The National Academies Press.

IOM (Institute of Medicine). 2003. *Health professions education: A bridge to quality.* Washington, DC: The National Academies Press.

IOM. 2004. *Keeping patients safe: Transforming the work environment of nurses.* Washington, DC: The National Academies Press.

Leape, L. L., A. G. Lawthers, T. A. Brennan, and W. G. Johnson. 1993. Preventing medical injury. *QRB Quality Review Bulletin* 19(5):144-149.

Maxfield, D., J. Grenny, R. McMillan, K. Patterson, and A. Switzler. 2005. *Silence kills: The seven crucial conversations for healthcare.* Provo, UT: VitalSmarts. Available at: http://www.silencekills.com (accessed February 24, 2010).

McCarthy, D., S. K. H. How, C. Schoen, J. C. Cantor, and D. Belloff. 2009. *Aiming higher: Results from a state scorecard on health system performance, 2009.* New York: The Commonwealth Fund.

Mitchell, P. H., S. Armstrong, T. F. Simpson, and M. Lentz. 1989. American Association of Critical-Care Nurses demonstration project: Profile of excellence in critical care nursing. *Heart & Lung: The Journal of Critical Care* 18(3):219-237.

Mitchell, P. H., S. E. Shannon, K. C. Cain, and S. T. Hegyvary. 1996. Critical care outcomes: Linking structures, processes, and organizational and clinical outcomes. *American Journal of Critical Care* 5(5):353-363; quiz 364-365.

Mitchell, P. H., B. Belza, D. C. Schaad, L. S. Robins, F. J. Gianola, P. S. Odegard, D. Kartin, and R. A. Ballweg. 2006. Working across the boundaries of health professions disciplines in education, research, and service: The University of Washington experience. *Academic Medicine* 81(10):891-896.

Rosenstein, A. H. 2002. Original research: Nurse–physician relationships: Impact on nurse satisfaction and retention. *American Journal of Nursing* 102(6):26-34.

Rosenstein, A. H. 2009. Early intervention can help prevent disruptive behavior. *Physician Executive* 35(6):14-15.

Rosenstein, A. H., and M. O'Daniel. 2005. Disruptive behavior and clinical outcomes: Perceptions of nurses and physicians. *American Journal of Nursing* 105(1):54-64; quiz 64-65.

Rosenstein, A. H., and M. O'Daniel. 2006. Impact and implications of disruptive behavior in the perioperative arena. *Journal of the American College of Surgeons* 203(1):96-105.

Rosenstein, A. H., and M. O'Daniel. 2008a. Invited article: Managing disruptive physician behavior: Impact on staff relationships and patient care. *Neurology* 70(17):1564-1570.

Rosenstein, A. H., and M. O'Daniel. 2008b. A survey of the impact of disruptive behaviors and communication defects on patient safety.

Joint Commission Journal of Quality and Patient Safety 34(8):464-471.

Rosenstein, A. H., H. Russell, and R. Lauve. 2002. Disruptive physician behavior contributes to nursing shortage. Study links bad behavior by doctors to nurses leaving the profession. *Physician Executive* 28(6):8-11.

RWJF and IHI (The Robert Wood Johnson Foundation and Institute for Healthcare Improvement). 2007. *Transforming care at the bedside: A new era in nursing.* Princeton, NJ, and Boston, MA: The Robert Wood Johnson Foundation and Institute for Healthcare Improvement.

Shaw, G. 2009. *Can health care quality improve and cost decrease? Pilot project in Atlantic City may show the way.* Princeton, NJ: Robert Wood Johnson Foundation.

Shortell, S. M., R. R. Gillies, D. A. Anderson, K. M. Erickson, and J. B. Mitchell. 1996. Remaking health care in America. *Hospitals & Health Networks* 70(6):43-44, 46, 48.

Tucker, A. L., and S. J. Spear. 2006. Operational failures and interruptions in hospital nursing. *Health Services Research* 41(3 Pt 1):643-662.

Wenzel, R. P., and M. B. Edmond. 2001. The impact of hospital-acquired bloodstream infections. *Emerging Infectious Diseases* 7(2):174-177.

B

Agenda

Forum on the Future of Nursing: Acute Care

Harvey Morse Auditorium
Cedars-Sinai Medical Center
8700 Beverly Boulevard, Los Angeles, CA 90048

October 19, 2009

AGENDA

12:30 pm   **Welcome and Introductions**
Linda Burnes Bolton, Cedars-Sinai Medical Center
Tom Priselac, Cedars-Sinai Medical Center

1:00 pm   **Acute Care: Current and Future State**
Marilyn Chow, Kaiser Permanente

1:30 pm   **Panel on Quality and Safety**
Maureen Bisognano, Institute for Healthcare
* Improvement*
Tami Minnier, University of Pittsburgh Medical
* Center*

Reactor Panel
Bernice Coleman, Cedars-Sinai Medical Center
Nancy Chiang, California Student Nurses
  Association
Kurt Swartout, Kaiser Permanente
Joseph Guglielmo, University of California–San
  Francisco
Julia Hallisy, The Empowered Patient Coalition

Committee Q&A and Discussion

2:15 pm   **Break**

2:30 pm   **Panel on Technology**
Steve DeMello, Public Health Institute
Pam Cipriano, University of Virginia Health System

Reactor Panel

Committee Q&A and Discussion

3:15 pm   **Panel on Interdisciplinary Collaboration**
Alan Rosenstein, VHA West Coast
Pamela Mitchell, University of Washington

Reactor Panel

Committee Q&A and Discussion

4:00 pm   **Presentation of Testimony**

5:25 pm   **Closing Remarks**
Josef Reum, The George Washington University

5:30 pm   **Forum Adjourns**

C

Speaker Biosketches

Maureen Bisognano, B.S.N., M.S.N., executive vice president and COO, Institute for Healthcare Improvement (IHI), is responsible for the day-to-day management of the Institute's many programs designed to improve health care delivery. Ms. Bisognano oversees all operations, program development, and strategic planning for the Institute. She also advises senior leaders around the world on improving healthcare systems. Ms. Bisognano is on the faculty of the Harvard School of Public Health and a member of the Commonwealth Fund's Commission on a High Performance Health System. Prior to joining IHI, she served as CEO of the Massachusetts Respiratory Hospital and senior vice president of The Juran Institute.

Linda Burnes Bolton, Dr.P.H., R.N., FAAN, is vice chair, Robert Wood Johnson Foundation (RWJF) Initiative on the Future of Nursing, at the Institute of Medicine. Dr. Burnes Bolton is vice president for Nursing, chief nursing officer, and director of Nursing Research at Cedars-Sinai Medical Center in Los Angeles. She is one of the Principal Investigators at the Cedars-Sinai Burns & Allen Research Institute. Her research, teaching, and clinical expertise includes nursing and patient care outcomes research, performance improvement, and improving the quality of care and cultural diversity within the health professions. She served as the national advisory chair for Transforming Care at the Bedside, an initiative of RWJF, to improve the nursing practice environment. Dr. Burnes Bolton is a past president of the American Academy of Nursing and the National Black Nurses Association.

Nancy Chiang, R.N., B.S.N., is a recent graduate from California State University, Sacramento. She was an active participant in the National Student Nurses' Association throughout her nursing education. On the chapter level, she held board positions during all 3 years of the program. From October 2008 through October 2009, Ms. Chiang served as secretary/treasurer for the California Nursing Students' Association. She believes her involvement with the Nursing Students' Association better prepared her for her position as a professional nurse on the Trauma Nursing Unit at the University of California–Davis Medical Center in Sacramento.

Marilyn P. Chow, D.N.Sc., R.N., FAAN, is the vice president, Patient Care Services, Program Office, at Kaiser Permanente. She is also the program director for the RWJF Executive Nurse Fellows Program. A graduate of the University of California–San Francisco (UCSF) School of Nursing, Dr. Chow has made significant contributions to nursing throughout her scholarship, leadership, and political and civic involvement. She is recognized for her expertise in leadership, innovation, regulation of nursing practice, workforce policy, and primary care. Her career has focused on promoting the role of nurses in primary care, advanced practice, and hospital-based care. She has coauthored four books, including the award-winning *Handbook of Pediatric Primary Care*. She is the co-principal investigator for the national study *How Do Medical–Surgical Nurses Spend Their Time?* She has received several awards, including the Women's Honors in Public Health and the UCSF School of Nursing Distinguished Alumni Award. She was recently selected as one of the distinguished 100 graduates and faculty of the UCSF School of Nursing for the Centennial Wall of Fame.

Pamela Cipriano, Ph.D., R.N., FAAN, recently completed 9 years as the chief nursing officer at the University of Virginia Medical Center, achieving Magnet Recognition. Dr. Cipriano chairs the American Academy of Nursing's Workforce Commission, studying technology solutions to improve the work environment to make patient care safer and more efficient. She serves as editor-in-chief of *American Nurse Today*, the official journal of the American Nurses Association. Throughout her career, she has been a leader in national nursing organizations addressing issues of policy, administration, quality, and clinical practice. She serves on The Joint Commission's National Nursing Advisory Council. She has been a Sigma Theta Tau International Distinguished Scholar and an American Nurses Foundation Scholar.

Bernice Coleman, Ph.D., ACNP-BC FAHA, has 25 combined years of advanced-practice nursing experience as a clinical nurse specialist. She is currently a board-certified acute care nurse practitioner in the Heart Transplantation and Ventricular Assist Programs at Cedars-Sinai Medical Center in Los Angeles. Her research area has focused on translational bench explorations of the clinical ethnic impact of cytokine gene polymorphisms on heart transplantation outcomes. Dr. Coleman has presented and published on the topics associated with care of the cardiac surgical patient, critical care nursing issues, and ethnic immunogenetics of heart transplantation. She was recently awarded the 2008 Distinguished Alumna Award from the Yale School of Nursing and the GE Healthcare and American Association of Critical-Care Nurses 2009 Pioneering Spirit Award in 2009. She is a volunteer faculty member in the Department of Physiology at UCSF, where she is mentoring and lecturing students in clinical genetics.

Steven DeMello, M.B.A., has more than 30 years of experience in research, hospital operations, strategic planning, systems management and consulting. He is currently the director of Health Care for the Center for Information Technology Research in the Interest of Society (CITRIS) at the University of California–Berkeley. Prior to joining CITRIS, he was executive director and senior advisor of the Health Technology Center (HealthTech), a nonprofit research group and expert network based in San Francisco. Prior to HealthTech, he served as chief operating officer of ezboard, Inc., a large first generation consumer social networking company. His previous positions include serving as senior vice president of the California Healthcare System, president and COO of Alliance Home Care Management, Inc., and principal at the global management consulting firm A.T. Kearney. He received a B.A. in economics from Claremont McKenna College and an M.B.A. from the University of Chicago.

Joseph Guglielmo, Pharm.D., is professor and chair of the Department of Clinical Pharmacy at the UCSF School of Pharmacy. In addition, he serves as associate director of Pharmaceutical Services for the UCSF Medical Center and director of the Department of Clinical Pharmacy Medication Outcomes Center. He is responsible for all evidence-based reviews and medication use evaluations at the medical center. The developer of the UCSF Antimicrobial Management Program, he also serves as infectious diseases pharmacist for UCSF Medical Center. His research interests center on the appropriate use of antimicrobials and acute care pharmacy practice models. Dr. Guglielmo is a long-term editor of *Applied Therapeutics* and the *Handbook of Applied Therapeutics* and a frequent contributor to healthcare professional journals.

Julia Hallisy, D.D.S., is a practicing dentist in San Francisco. In 1989, Dr. Hallisy's late daughter, Katherine, was born with bilateral retinoblastoma. Dealing with Kate's life-threatening diagnosis, the many recurrences of cancer, and the unanticipated challenges of hospital-acquired infection and misdiagnosis gave Dr. Hallisy valuable insight as an advocate for patients. The many lessons she learned during Kate's life became the foundation for her book, *The Empowered Patient: Hundreds of Life-Saving Facts, Action Steps and Strategies You Need to Know.* Dr. Hallisy is committed to and passionate about the subjects of patient safety, healthcare reform, and medical error reduction. Her personal and professional goals include working diligently to help give patients a voice in healthcare solutions. Dr. Hallisy has most recently worked with another advocate, Helen Haskell, in forming The Empowered Patient Coalition nonprofit organization.

Tamra (Tami) E. Minnier, R.N., M.S.N., FACHE, is the chief quality officer for the University of Pittsburgh Medical Center (UPMC). The mission of the Center for Quality Improvement and Innovation is to partner with hospital leadership to change care delivery systems in support of the UPMC vision of creating the health system of the future. Ms. Minnier has studied the Toyota Production System, Lean Manufacturing, and other business improvement applications to health care. A nationally known speaker, Ms. Minnier has been published in several articles. She received her B.S.N. and M.S.N. from the University of Pittsburgh.

Pamela H. Mitchell, Ph.D., R.N., FAHA, FAAN, is professor of Biobehavioral Nursing and Health Systems; associate dean for Research, School of Nursing; adjunct professor, Department of Health Services; and founding director of the Center for Health Sciences Interprofessional Education and Research at the University of Washington. Her research and teaching focus on hospital care delivery systems, effective management of clinical care systems, biobehavioral interventions for patients with acute and chronic cardio-cerebrovascular disease, and outcomes of interprofessional education. These works are funded by the National Institute of Nursing; National Heart, Lung, and Blood Institute; Bureau of Health Professions, Health Resources and Services Administration; and the Josiah Macy, Jr. Foundation. She is president of the American Academy of Nursing and is a member and past chair of the Expert Panel on Quality Healthcare. She is immediate past chair, Nursing and Rehabilitation Professionals Committee, Stroke Council of the American Heart/American Stroke Association.

Thomas M. Priselac, is president and CEO of the Cedars-Sinai Health System, a position he has held since 1994. Mr. Priselac has been associated with Cedars-Sinai since 1979. Prior to his current position, he was executive vice president from 1988 to 1993. Before joining Cedars-Sinai, he was on the executive staff of Montefiore Hospital in Pittsburgh. He currently serves as chair of the American Hospital Association Board of Trustees. He is a past chair of the Association of American Medical Colleges. He currently serves on the Los Angeles Chamber of Commerce Board, where he previously chaired the Health Care Committee. He formerly chaired the Hospital Association of Southern California, the California Healthcare Association, and the Association of American Medical Colleges Council of Teaching Hospitals. Mr. Priselac is an author and invited speaker on a variety of contemporary issues facing health care today, including policy issues related to the delivery and financing of health care, healthcare quality and safety, and the adoption and implementation of information technology.

Josef Reum, Ph.D., is the interim dean of the School of Public Health and Health Services at the George Washington University (GWU). Prior to joining the GWU faculty in 1993, Dr. Reum was CEO of the American Health Quality Association, which represents organizations that provide evaluation and quality improvement services to healthcare purchasers and providers. His administrative skills were also essential to his tasks as deputy director of the Local Initiative Funding Partners Program, an RWJF national program designed to promote innovation in the design and delivery of healthcare services. Dr. Reum has held leadership positions in six states, including commissioner of the Department of Mental Health, Developmental Disabilities and Substance Abuse (Indiana), deputy commissioner of the Department of Mental Retardation (Massachusetts), and director of the Anchorage Department of Health and Social Services (Alaska).

Alan Rosenstein, M.D., M.B.A., is currently vice president and medical director for VHA West Coast, Pleasanton, California, and medical director for Physician Wellness Services, Minneapolis. He is the former vice president of Clinical Informatics for McKesson-HBOC, former medical director of Decision Support for HBSI-Solucient, and former director of Medical Resource Management and manager of Outcome Measurement at California Pacific Medical Center in San Francisco. He has also served as medical director for several regional managed care organizations. He graduated from the University of Louisville School of Medicine. He completed his internship at Highland General Hospital in Oakland, California, and 3 years of residency in Internal Medicine at Mount Zion Hospital and Medical Center in San Francisco. He has more than 100 publications and numerous lectures, seminar presentations, and national and international consultation experiences in the areas of performance improvement, information management, decision support, performance profiling, health economics, resource and case management, technology assessment, outcomes analysis, nurse–physician relationships, organizational dynamics, physician engagement and leadership, patient safety, quality improvement, and cost-effective care. He earned his M.B.A. in Health Services Management at Golden Gate University in San Francisco.

Kurt Swartout, M.D., following his medical residency, joined the Permanente Medical Group and worked in primary care for 2 years before transitioning into its hospitalist program. As a hospitalist, Dr. Swartout specializes in the care of hospitalized patients as well as adult patients with medical problems in the emergency department. He especially enjoys meeting patients in the emergency department, formulating a plan, and getting the patients well enough so they can return home. Dr. Swartout is a member of the American College of Physicians and Kaiser Permanente's Palliative Care Service, which provides patient and family education for patients whose disease is not responding to curative treatment. He has served as chief of Hospital Medicine at Kaiser Roseville since 1999, and he has been an active participant in the Transforming Care at the Bedside program since 2003. Dr. Swartout received his M.D. from the University of California–Davis School of Medicine in 1991, and completed his internship and residency at the university's Medical Center in 1994.